Understanding Your Pet's Lab Work

A Guide to Communicating with your Veterinarian

Sally Suttenfield, DVM

UNDERSTANDING YOUR PET'S LAB WORK

Print edition. February 5, 2023

ISBN: 9798395192110

Written by Sally Suttenfield, DVM

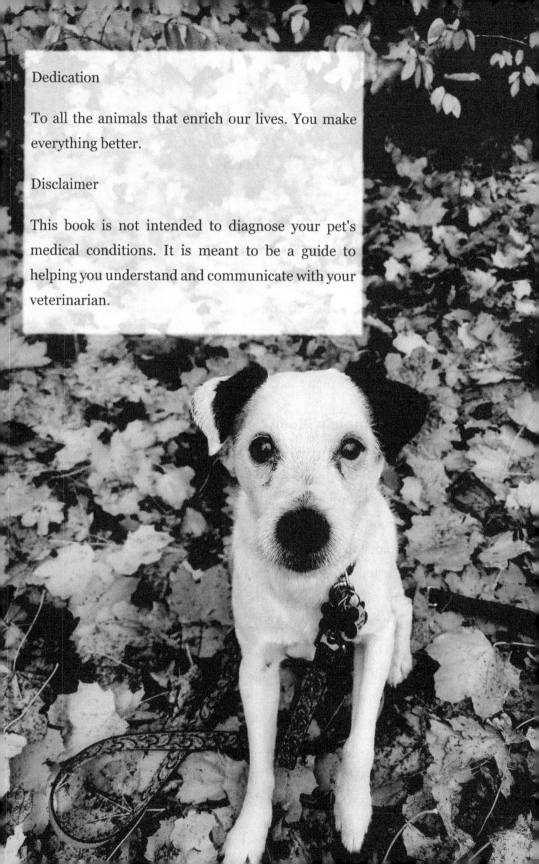

Dedication

To all the animals that enrich our lives. You make everything better.

Disclaimer

This book is not intended to diagnose your pet's medical conditions. It is meant to be a guide to helping you understand and communicate with your veterinarian.

Contents

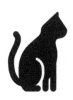

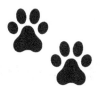

Introduction

You've just been handed a copy of your dog's lab work, and your vet zeroes in on a few key points. Other values, highs and lows alike, seem to be ignored. Why?

Perhaps your vet has ordered a whole battery of tests for your cat. Are they all necessary? If finances dictated that you choose some tests and eliminate others, could you do so?

CBC with differential. Chem panel. Urinalysis via cystocentesis. Some of these phrases may sound familiar to you from watching medical dramas on television. How much do you, as a pet owner, need to know?

You need to know enough to be able to make informed decisions about the well-being of your pet. The objective of this book is not to replace communication with your veterinarian but to provide the basic information necessary to help you decide how to proceed when your pet is ill. Understanding the basics is crucial to appreciating the need for certain tests, as well as their limitations.

Many veterinarians, fresh out of school, are cautioned against providing lengthy explanations for fear of overwhelming their clients with too much information. Many clients are reluctant to ask for more detailed information. This text is designed to be a bridge between the two.

Why Write This Book?

I'm a small-town veterinarian who likes to talk. I *like* explaining things. Everyone deserves to get the information available to make the best possible decisions when it comes to deciding what to do next with a sick pet or how to keep them well in the first place. The material in this book is the same information I relay to my clients when discussing their pet's lab work findings.

I also wrote this book for all the intelligent, discerning pet lovers out there who want to understand the implications behind the test results they are given. From my earliest days as a freshly minted graduate, I've been told not to confuse the clientele by "information-overload."

"They don't need to know all that stuff," one former boss told me. "Just tell them what's wrong and what they need to do about it."

What I heard from clients was quite different. Time and again people tell me that no one has ever explained to them what was going on with their dog or cat in such detail. "I wish my own doctor would tell me as much about *me*," one client said to me.

So, this book is intended to fill that gap.

How to Use This Book

What makes this book different is that I explain the *why* behind the bare facts of the test results.

This really is not intended as some sort of "first aid" type book. Oh sure, you can quickly check for the definition of BUN after it comes up in a discussion with your veterinarian, but in an emergency, the information in this book may be too dense to digest rapidly. This information is best used in one of two ways: as background material against future situations or for learning more after a diagnosis has been made.

If you are a "don't tell me why" person, you will want to skip over the in-depth explanations of the workings of a red blood cell or the sources of certain serum enzymes. That's okay. You can cut to the chase with the **NEWSFLASH** points that come with certain sections.

But I believe the *why* of lab work to be particularly important. If you are one of those people who thoroughly researches all your options online after every vet visit, then the information provided here might help you decode some of the articles you are reading. However, the main reason for reading this book is to understand what the lab work you've been given means. You may not be given the data itself. You may simply be told, your dog has "X" problem. Do you know how to interpret that? What are the implications? What's the prognosis? My goal with this book is to give you the tools to better understand the information that you've been given—if nothing else, so you can ask the right questions.

Section 1: The Minimum Database

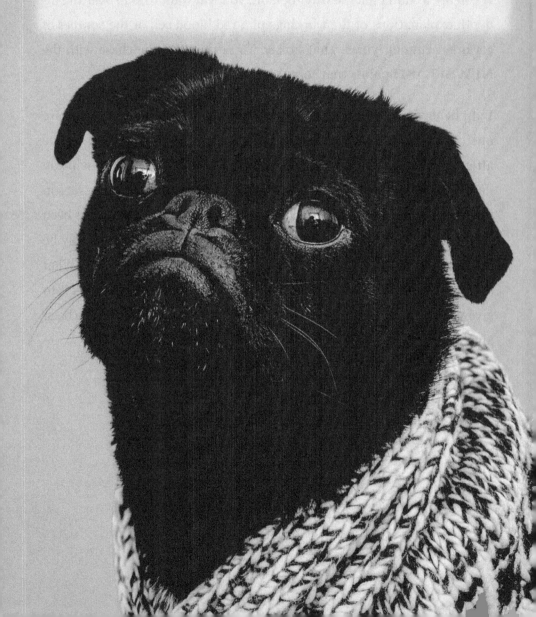

The Minimum Database

When you come into the vet clinic with a sick dog or cat, and it's not clear what's going on, your veterinarian has a variety of tests available to help identify the underlying problem. If you have a healthy, older pet, and you request a senior exam, then your veterinarian may suggest running slightly different tests. If you have an animal with some chronic health issues (perhaps taking a wide variety of medications), another set of tests may be more appropriate. Many of the basic tests will be the same in all three cases, however.

Veterinarians refer to this basic set of tests as the **minimum database or MDB.**

What exactly is a *minimum database*? Simply put, this is a group of the most basic laboratory tests to screen for common health problems in your pet. It's the starting point for any animal that comes in with an illness of unknown cause, an animal with vague symptoms, or an animal with an appointment for a routine health screening. If a specific problem is suspected, then the type and number of tests may be modified, but the MDB is a set of core tests performed to consistently achieve an accurate diagnosis of your pet's condition. It allows your vet to build a picture of illness or health.

In general, the MDB will consist of a complete blood cell count (CBC), a serum chemistry panel, electrolyte levels, a urinalysis, a fecal float for intestinal parasites, and in some cases, heartworm testing (and possibly feline leukemia/FIV testing for cats). If some of these tests have been performed recently, or if your pet is taking heartworm prevention regularly, some of these tests might be optional. We will examine each of these components in turn and determine what it can or can't tell us.

For the purposes of avoiding the phrase "dog or cat" repeatedly, you can assume that any information here is also applicable to cats—unless I say otherwise. Cats are not small dogs, however! They are a distinct species with different metabolic needs, so there will be more on the unique attributes of cats later.

If you take your dog to the vet with an ear infection, do you really need a MDB to determine what the problem is? The answer is "that depends." A simple, uncomplicated **otitis** (ear infection) may need only a microscopic examination of an ear swab to determine the cause. If, however, your dog has chronic, severe ear problems, your work-up may include an MDB, as well as an ear culture and specific testing for allergies or hypothyroidism. Your veterinarian will help you decide when such testing is warranted, but do not be afraid to ask for testing if you feel it will be beneficial in reaching a solution for your pet's health problems. Remember information is power!

What does a MDB usually consist of?

- CBC

- Serum chemistry profile

- Urinalysis

- Fecal

- Heartworm test (and/or FeLV/FIV test)

When is a MDB performed?

- Whenever you have a sick pet

- Any pet with unexplained weight loss

- Any pet with excessive water consumption/urination

- A pet about to undergo an anesthetic procedure

- Annually or semi-annually on dogs or cats over eight years old

Section 2: The Complete Blood Count

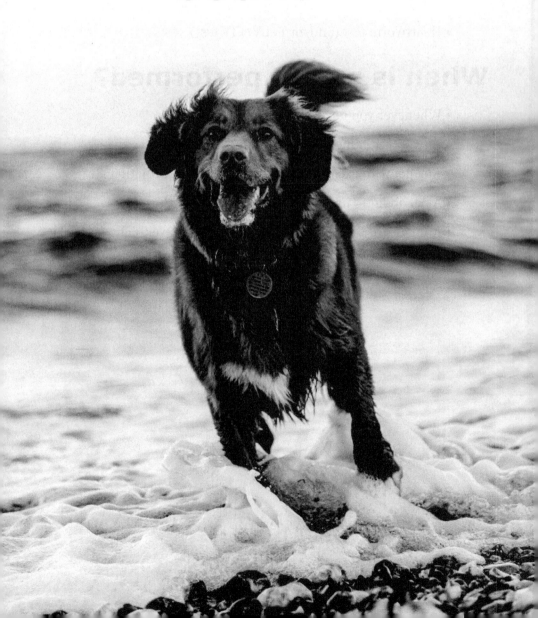

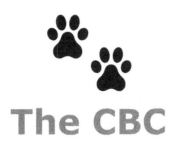

The CBC

"CBC" stands for **complete blood count.** It looks at the total numbers of red cells, white cells, and platelets carried in a fluid called plasma circulating in your dog's bloodstream.

- The red cells carry oxygen and other important products throughout the body.

- The white cells fight infection and develop antibodies in response to anything that challenges the immune system. The way in which the white cell numbers respond to a problem can help identify the presence of certain types of infections or inflammatory reactions, such as allergies.

- Platelets help prevent and stop bleeding after an injury.

A **differential** is a description of the breakdown on the numbers of red cells, platelets, individual white cell types, and their proportions to each other, as well as a look at cell **morphology** (appearance and structure). In other words—what are the blood cells doing and are they happy?

If the blood sample is sent to an outside laboratory for testing, then most of the time, a differential is performed even if the vet does not specifically request or need it. It's just standard practice. If your vet has a testing machine in house, these are now capable of distinguishing one cell type from another, but not all in-house machines can determine cell morphology. Unless trained personnel examine a blood smear under a microscope, that specific kind of information might not be determined.

So, let's take a little crash course in examining the CBC and defining some of the terms. Now don't panic. If you're like me and your eyes glaze over at the thought of looking at charts and graphs before you have even had a chance to familiarize yourself with the terms, then you can skip this part and come back to it after you have read over the text. That is the beauty of a manual like this. Unlike a novel, you aren't going to lose out on important information if you skip around a little. You can always come back later! As a vet student, I had large volumes of information thrown at me in rapid succession. I learned then a striking metaphor for life: the important stuff gets repeated. Repeat after me, the important stuff gets repeated.

The first thing to keep in mind when looking at a copy of some lab work is that every lab or piece of lab equipment is going to have its own way of presenting the information. Overall, the basic information will be the same, but the way the information is displayed will vary depending on who is reporting the data. Some lab profiles only focus on key test results and may leave out certain pieces of information altogether. Think of it like the national nightly news on television. Different networks are going to put their own spin on the major breaking stories in the world. In this case, your focus should be on what the story is about, and you should worry less about how it is told.

That said, here is an example of what a CBC might look like, carried out on my own dog, Abbey, as part of a routine senior exam. At the time, she was a 9-year-old, spayed, German Shepherd.

Test Requested	Results	Reference Range	Units
Hemoglobin (Hb)	17.1	12.1-20.3	g/dl
Hematocrit (HCT)	50.3	33-45	%
WBC	4.4	4-15.5	$10^3/\mu l$
RBC	7.29	4.8-9.3	$10^3/\mu l$
MCV	71	58-79	
MCH	23.1	19-28	
MCHC	32.3	30-384	
Platelet count (PLT)	192	170-400	$10^3/\mu l$
Platelet estimate	adequate	adequate	
Reticulocytes	0 %	(Elevation here is significant)	

Differential	Absolute	%	Reference Range
Neutrophils	2772	63	2060-10600
Bands	0	0	0-300
Lymphocytes	748	17	690-4500
Monocytes	440	10	0-840
Eosinophils	440	10	0-1200
Basophils	0	0	0-150

Wow. Looks a little intimidating, doesn't it? If you've never looked at a CBC report before, it might not make much sense to you. So, let's look quickly at each line and column before delving into the figures themselves. The four columns first:

COLUMN 1 – what's being measured and tested

COLUMN 2 – your dog's results – the numbers you'll learn to understand

COLUMN 3 – reference ranges. These are the readings I'd expect to see for a normal, healthy animal of the same age as the one we're testing.

Normal ranges on lab tests can vary with the age of the animal as well as the species, so it is advisable to run the bloodwork on a system that can account for these differences if possible. Each lab will provide its own reference ranges of normal test results.

Although the reports from different labs will have the same basic characteristics, they may have some slight differences in the way the information is reported. *Ignore those differences*: it is beyond the scope of this book to delve that deeply into the technical aspects of laboratory testing, and we will just get bogged down in trivial details. The important thing is to compare your pet's results to the normal range provided for those laboratory tests.

COLUMN 4: the units of measurement for each assay

Now let's look in detail at COLUMN 1 and see what each test does:

**Test
Requested**

Hemoglobin (Hb)	A protein inside red blood cells that transports oxygen
Hematocrit (HCT)	The percentage of red cells in your total blood volume
WBC	White blood cell count
RBC	Red blood cell count

**Test
Requested**

MCV **MCH** **MCHC**	These are terms used to describe red cell morphology — that is, their size, shape, and color. This information is beyond the scope of this text. For that reason, we won't delve into it any further in this text.
Platelet count (PLT)	Pieces of megakaryocytes from the bone marrow that help form blood clots and slow down bleeding
Platelet estimate	A rough estimate of the total platelet numbers as opposed to an actual count
Reticulocytes	Level of immature, 'baby" red cells found. Any number above zero is a cause for further investigation.

Differential

Neutrophils	A type of white blood cells that forms a major defense in fighting infection

Differential

Bands	Immature neutrophils
Lymphocytes	A type of immune cell found in the blood and lymphatic tissue
Monocytes	A type of white blood cell that fights germs (viruses, bacteria, fungi, and protozoa) and eliminates infected cells
Eosinophils	A type of white blood cell most commonly activated when there is a parasitic infection, an allergic reaction, or cancer
Basophils	Least common white blood cell, important in early detection of some kinds of cancer and in some allergic responses

So, now that you know what's being tested, what does a CBC really tell us? Mostly, it looks at the relative numbers of red cells and white cells circulating in the bloodstream, among other things. The CBC is best understood if we look at the red cells and white cells separately.

Section 2.1: Red Blood Cells and Anemia

The average life span of a red blood cell is 120 days. After that time, they naturally degrade and are replaced. Healthy bone marrow produces a steady supply of new red and white cells all the time.

When we describe a pet as having anemia, what we mean is their red cell count is too low. There are several different ways of making this assessment. Most lab machines perform an actual red cell count, expressed in so many million cells per microliter of blood. Sometimes, your vet may refer to indirect measurements, such as the hematocrit (HCT) or PCV. These are just terms to indicate the technique used to determine the information. PCV stands for *packed cell volume* and looks at the **percentage of red cells** verses the total blood volume after it has been spun in a *hematocrit* tube that separates the red cells from the liquid volume of blood. A lab might refer to either the PCV or the HCT, but they are the same thing. What is important is whether the PCV too low or too high when compared to normal ranges.

When the PCV is low, it's showing a deficiency of red cells. In other words, **a low PCV may indicate anemia.** Picture a fish tank filled with water and fish gravel. The water equals the "plasma," and the gravel equals the "packed red blood cells." If you have very little gravel relative to the amount of water in the tank, you might be anemic.

Because the red cells circulate oxygen, an animal that is anemic can often show signs of respiratory distress. Sometimes weakness and difficulty breathing might be the first thing you as a pet owner will see. This is because **hemoglobin** (HGB) molecules within the red blood cells carry oxygen throughout the blood stream, and HGB levels will be low if your pet is anemic. Decreased numbers of red blood cells mean decreased opportunities for HGB to catch a ride through the blood stream. Plus, if your red cells are being lost or destroyed, the same thing will happen to your hemoglobin, too.

An anemic cat may breathe with its mouth open. **Open-mouthed breathing is never normal in a cat!** The cat is either stressed/frightened or not getting enough oxygen for whatever reason. This is a **medical emergency** and requires immediate contact with your veterinarian. If you've been playing with your cat, and he begins to pant, stop play and let him calm down. If he doesn't begin breathing normally in a short period of time, then contact your vet.

An animal can become anemic from several causes, but the mechanism of anemia boils down to one of two problems. Either blood is being lost at a greater rate than it can be replaced (e.g., acute blood loss or hemorrhage due to accident or a condition such as autoimmune hemolytic anemia, worms, etc.) or the blood cells are undergoing natural attrition (dying off from old age), but new cells aren't being made to replace them.

In other words, if you make regular deposits to your bank account, but spend more money than you deposit because of some big expenses, you overdraw your account due to excessive loss, just like blood loss anemia or hemolytic anemia (see more on these below). On the other hand, if your spending habits are not excessive, but you stop making deposits to your account, you will still eventually overdraw your account. This is the equivalent of anemia due to lack of replacement cells. You can see where lack of replacement due to lack of incoming funds might be a harder problem to correct. It's easier to find and stop the source of excessive loss than it is to find funds that don't exist.

In the face of anemia, the correct response by the bone marrow is to increase production of the blood cells. So, after an animal is diagnosed with anemia, we look closely at the blood cells to determine if the anemia is **regenerative** or **non-regenerative.** We're asking the question: is this animal trying to compensate for the anemia by generating new red blood cells (**regenerative** anemia) or not (**non-regenerative** anemia)? We need this information because the answer might help determine both the cause and the prognosis.

This is where cell morphology comes into play—now we're looking at what the cells look like. The size and shape of the red cell can sometimes help determine the source of the anemia, such as the presence of spherocytes in cases of anemia caused by autoimmune illness (**autoimmune hemolytic anemia -AIHA**). We examine what the cell looks like by looking at the MCV, MCH, and MCHC results and the presence and level of reticulocytes (see below) when the blood is examined under a microscope.

(In addition, blood parasites, toxic changes, or evidence of immune destruction can be seen when the blood smear is examined microscopically.)

Regenerative Anemia

A regenerative anemia indicates that the body *recognizes* that it is anemic and has increased the production of new red blood cells in the bone marrow—to the point of releasing immature red blood cells called

reticulocytes or **nucleated red blood cells,** which can be seen under a microscope. Reticulocytes are "baby" red blood cells. Their presence usually indicates that the demand for new red cells is so great that immature cells are being kicked out into circulation before they are fully developed.

Remember the table of lab results we saw above? Here's a reminder of the relevant lines:

Test Requested

RBC	Red blood cell count
MCV	These are terms used to describe red cell morphology — that is, their size, shape, and color. This information is beyond the scope of this text. For that reason, we won't delve into it any further in this text.
MCH	
MCHC	
Reticulocytes	Immature, "baby" red cells. Any number above zero is a cause for further investigation.

In general, anemias due to loss of blood tend to be regenerative. A **strongly** regenerative anemia is more likely due to **hemolysis** (abnormal destruction of red blood cells by the body) rather than blood loss through an accident that results in heavy bleeding or blood loss through parasites. Because the red cells are being destroyed in a hemolytic anemia, the contents of the red cells are released into the blood stream, so all the components to make new red cells are *still available* for the body to use again. That means it is easier to make more red blood cells in this situation because all the bits are still there. In anemia due to blood loss, however, the cellular components are lost to use (because they have completely left the body), and the body must then make new red cells from scratch. That is a bigger drain on the system and is more likely to result in shortages.

If the red cell numbers have dropped rapidly (such as acute blood loss from trauma), there may be a delay before the PCV reflects the true value. The body will do everything it can to compensate for blood loss in an emergency. It will close blood supply to less critical areas and redirect resources to compensate for the losses. At some point, however, the loss of blood will have a visible effect. Sudden drops in PCV values are harder to compensate for than a gradual decline (say, from a fleabite anemia). This means if your dog has lost a lot of blood due to an injury, values higher than the 12% typically required for transfusion may still be life-threatening. **The important lesson here is that slow, gradual blood-loss is better tolerated and harder for you as the owner to identify!**

Until oxygen-carrying capacity is affected, the only thing that you might notice with slow blood loss in your anemic pet is a decrease in activity. Difficulty breathing, pale mucus membranes, or a rapid respiratory rate can indicate severe anemia.

Non-regenerative anemia

A non-regenerative anemia, where the body doesn't seem to be compensating by producing immature red cells, can indicate that the anemia might not be severe enough to trigger a bone marrow response. Many geriatric animals are mildly anemic. This isn't necessarily a cause for concern. But a non-regenerative anemia can also indicate that the body has exhausted its stores, either because of excessive loss or because it is incapable of mounting a response in the first place. If the bone marrow can't ramp up production to make new red blood cells, then as the old cells die off, they won't be replaced. A non-regenerative anemia can sometimes indicate a serious underlying problem, like cancer. If an animal is severely anemic, and the anemia is not regenerative, then the prognosis is guarded. The body should be working as hard as it can to counterbalance the anemia.

That makes sense, right? If there is a shortage of products in the grocery store, the chance of getting something you need is better if the farmers and the producers are working overtime to get supplies to the store. But if the farmers are wiped out by drought (or a pandemic), then there is nothing coming down the line to the store. The shelves are bare.

A non-responsive or non-regenerative anemia means that the bone marrow is not compensating for the low red blood cell count by increasing its output. This is likely to happen with chronic diseases, such as kidney dysfunction, with some drug therapies that suppress the bone marrow, some types of immune-mediated diseases, and some forms of cancer. Non-regeneration usually indicates that the problem will be harder to correct. A severely depleted red blood cell "bank account" in combination with lack of regeneration is of grave concern. The cause of the anemia must be determined and corrected if possible.

One of the hormones that signals the bone marrow to release new red blood cells is **erythropoietin**. This hormone is produced by the kidneys and often decreases with advanced kidney disease. Some kidney failure patients are placed on artificial or synthetic erythropoietin when their PCV drops below 20%. The bone marrow can be affected by certain chemotherapy agents, so sometimes you will hear of erythropoietin being prescribed in those cases, too.

General points on anemia

Profound anemia can cause spurious (fake) or exaggerated heart murmurs. When the blood is thinner, it becomes more turbulent as it travels through the heart, enhancing existing murmurs or creating murmurs where none existed before. If your pet is diagnosed with a heart murmur while anemic, it is important to follow up on the murmur once the anemia has been corrected. It may not be there anymore; if it is, further work up, such as an echocardiogram, is indicated.

Much more common is the borderline or low-grade anemia. Many times, your vet may not seem too concerned about this finding; quite often this is because many of the conditions that cause this type of anemia are self-correcting if the primary problem is resolved. Sometimes the underlying problem can only be managed rather than cured and a vitamin/mineral supplementation may be warranted. As we mentioned before, mild anemia may not be sufficient for the body to trigger a regenerative response.

A special mention of vitamin supplementation should be made here: over-supplementing with zinc can lead to an anemia that mimics an autoimmune hemolysis! This can take the form of excessive use of vitamins, an abnormal level of zinc in the food due to a manufacturer error, or from consuming pennies! If you have a young, otherwise healthy dog that develops severe anemia, and you've ruled out rat poison, be sure to rule out zinc toxicity as well!

Case Study: Ralphie, an example of anemia due to blood loss

Ralphie is a six-week-old puppy that lives outdoors in a dirt pen with his mother and littermates. He is heavily infested with fleas. His gums (**mucus membranes**) are very pale in color—almost white. He has not been vaccinated or dewormed. It is August in the mid-Atlantic region.

Here's Ralphie's CBC: Complete blood Count

Test Requested	Results	Reference Range	Units
Hemoglobin (Hb)	9.1 (**LOW**)	12.1-20.3	g/dl
Hematocrit (HCT)	15 (**LOW**)	33-45%	
WBC	4.4	4-15.5	$10^3/\mu l$
RBC	3.2 (**LOW**)	4.8-9.3	$10^3/\mu l$
Platelet count (PLT)	180	170-400	$10^3/\mu l$
Platelet estimate	Adequate	adequate	

Test Requested	Results	Reference Range	Units
Reticulocytes	3 % (any elevation here is significant)		

Differential	Absolute	%	Reference Range
Neutrophils	2772	63	2060-10600
Bands	0	0	0-300
Lymphocytes	388	7	690-4500
Eosinophils	800 ***	18 (H)	0-1200
Basophils	0	0	0-150

A hematocrit (**HCT or PCV**) of 15% indicates Ralphie is anemic. When the hematocrit or PCV values fall to **12% or below**, a blood transfusion is usually recommended. The low hemoglobin numbers are suggestive of blood loss - in this case to the fleas and parasites - as the hemoglobin is no longer available for the transmission of oxygen inside the red blood cell.

A 3% reticulocyte count is an indication of regeneration: Ralphie is trying to replace the blood cells that the fleas and parasites are taking! However, it is only a moderate effort. Diet and nutrition, as well as age, can play a role in how well the body responds to blood loss. If the problem has been going on for a while as well, then the body's resources may be tapped out.

Make note here of the relative increase in eosinophil numbers (marked with ***). Even though the overall number is still within normal limits, the percentage of eosinophils is high - a result often associated with parasites such as fleas or worms. We'll talk more about this later.

These values indicate that Ralphie is markedly anemic, possibly due to the fleas, but he should also be checked for intestinal parasites, particularly hookworms. In the Southeastern part of the United States, puppies can die from hookworm infections by six weeks of age if they have not been on a preventative deworming program. Dogs housed in pens with dirt floors are particularly susceptible to parasitic infection, as the parasite eggs thrive in damp soil. Not all parasites are worms, however! Protozoan parasites can also cause diarrhea and blood loss, so a fecal exam is highly recommended, even if there is a history of deworming. Unfortunately, parasite resistance is becoming more frequent, and despite a history of deworming, parasites can still be a cause of significant blood loss.

Ralphie should respond to flea control, deworming, and vitamin supplementation, but if his PCV were below 12%, he might need a blood transfusion to prevent kidney damage from decreased **renal** (kidney) blood flow. If he also has signs of pre-existing kidney dysfunction on his blood chemistry panel (more common in a geriatric animal but still possible), then this consideration becomes even more important.

Other causes of anemia need to be ruled out as well. Until the PCV improves or a blood transfusion is given, a pup this anemic must be handled very carefully during diagnosis and treatment. Too much stress before the anemia is corrected can kill such a medically fragile puppy. This fragility due to anemia may dictate treatment (and diagnostic testing) in stages rather than a whole battery of tests at one time.

Case Study: Muffy, an example of hemolytic anemia

Muffy is a six-year-old spayed female cocker spaniel. She has suddenly become lethargic, and on examination her gums appear yellow-tinged. Her temperature is 103.5 degrees Fahrenheit (normal temperature 101.5 to 102.5).

Muffy's CBC was performed on a typical in-house blood analysis machine. Because it determines the lab results in a different fashion from the first laboratory, the presentation of the material will look slightly different.

CBC:			**Reference Range**
HCT	14 %	**(LOW)**	37-55
HCB	3.7 g/dl	**(LOW)**	12-16
WBC	5.9 10⁹/L		6-16.9
NEUT	4.2 10⁹/L		2.8-10.5
EOS	0 10⁹/L		0.5-1.5

CBC:		Reference Range
Lymph/mono ratio (L/M)	1.7 10^9/L	1.1-6.5
PLT	180 10^9/L	175-500
Reticulocytes	8 % (elevated)	

This clinic machine does not report individual numbers for cell types, nor does it distinguish between lymphocytes and monocytes, reporting them as a single ratio. Most newer machines provide more detailed information, but this is an example of how things might look different. Remember, the details of presentation aren't as important as what the lab work tells us.

Muffy has a 14% red cell count with an 8% reticulocyte count. On microscopic examination of a blood smear, **spherocytes** are noted. Unlike normal red cells, spherocytes are missing some of the red cell membrane; they are like a soft pillow that's been stretched too tight by its cover—there is no "dent"—as there is in the center of a healthy red blood cell. These abnormal red blood cells indicate that Muffy is experiencing **autoimmune hemolytic anemia (AIHA)**. This is one of those times when having a trained lab tech look at the cell morphology is extremely helpful in making a diagnosis!

Muffy's body is destroying her own red blood cells because her immune system no longer *recognizes them as belonging to her*. The bone marrow is trying extremely hard to replace the destroyed cells but is not able to keep up with the losses. Emergency intervention with immunosuppressive drugs will be necessary to stop the cascade of destruction. The yellow tinge to her gums is a condition called **jaundice** (human term) or **icterus** (animal term). It is caused by the release of bilirubin from the destroyed red cells into her bloodstream. There are other causes of icterus besides AIHA, so any animal presenting with this sign needs a full workup.

AIHA is a severe, life-threatening disease with a guarded prognosis, even with aggressive treatment. Because AIHA has been associated with a recent history of certain kinds of vaccines, in general we don't recommend pets being treated for AIHA be vaccinated for anything but rabies (required by law) ever again. In some cases, it may be advisable for you to discuss with your vet whether even vaccinating for rabies is appropriate, but keep in mind, the law is not on your side when it comes to your pet's rabies status. The degree to which the law is enforced may vary with locality and the incidence of rabies in the immediate area.

Certain breeds of dogs and cats are more prone to auto-immune diseases, although AIHA is more common in dogs (particularly small, middle-aged, spayed females) than cats. Cocker spaniels are frequently affected. Other potentially susceptible breeds include poodles, Irish Setters, and Old English Sheepdogs. As we said before, in dogs it can be triggered by recent vaccination, but there are many triggers out there: insect bites, use of certain antibiotics or medications, stress...etc. An extremely rare trigger for AIHA is getting sprayed directly in the mouth by a skunk! So, if your dog gets skunked, consider having a CBC run about two weeks post-exposure. Most triggers do not cause clinical signs right away, but when a dog with a predisposition toward AIHA presents with certain clinical signs, your vet should be examining its recent history for such possible triggers—antibiotics, for instance—and avoid their use again in the future.

While cats are less likely to get AIHA, there seems to be a predisposition in the Somali breed. Also, AIHA in cats tends to be related to feline leukemia (a deadly virus in cats), a blood parasite called *Mycoplasma hemofelis*, or occasionally, it can be triggered by the medication methimazole, used to treat hyperthyroidism in geriatric cats.

But back to Missy's case: a chemistry profile would reveal some changes in Missy's bilirubin levels and liver enzymes. The combination of these changes in liver chemistries (which will be discussed later) plus the anemia indicate the damage is occurring from the abnormal destruction of the red cells as opposed to having a primary liver problem. The presence of the icterus also makes a condition such as autoimmune hemolytic anemia a much more likely cause of anemia than something like rat poisoning, which causes blood loss though an inability for the blood to clot normally. The elevated temperature is another feature common to autoimmune hemolytic anemia cases because the body is under tremendous stress. The fever is a result of the destruction of the red blood cells—this is an active, aggressive attack by Missy's immune system on her own body.

Should her red cell numbers continue to fall before the medication can start to suppress her overactive immune system, Muffy might need a blood transfusion to save her life. Her body will destroy the transfused blood rapidly as well, as it truly *will* be a foreign protein to her system. Transfusion with artificial blood products may work best in a case like this, as the artificial products cause fewer reactions. Bottom line, however, if a blood transfusion is needed to buy her time for the medications to kick in, then she should get one, ideally from a cross-matched donor. Unlike humans, dogs can tolerate a one-time donation from a non-matched donor in an emergency, where the availability of donors might be limited. But if your pet needs *repeated* transfusions, a blood-matched donor is best.

Can the PCV ever be too high?

Remember, that PCV stands for *packed cell volume* and looks at the **percentage of red cells** verses the total blood volume after it has been spun in a *hematocrit* tube that separates the red cells from the liquid volume of blood. Anemia, as we've seen, is indicated when the PCV is low compared to the reference range on the test. Should we worry when the PCV is higher than normal range?

Well, dehydration can decrease the amount of circulating plasma relative to the numbers of red blood cells. Picture the fish tank again. Now some of the "water" has been removed and it *seems* as though there is more "gravel" as a result. The red cell count itself hasn't changed, but the total amount of circulating fluid has. It is also important to keep in mind that if you have an anemic animal that is also dehydrated, then the dehydration will make the anemia seem less severe. Rehydration in the form of fluids, while necessary, will reveal the true degree of anemia. Sometimes a decision to perform a blood transfusion must be made after an animal is rehydrated.

Some species (mostly cats and horses but to a certain extent, dogs, too) may undergo **splenic contraction** during blood collection. The spleen, among other things, acts as a reservoir for RBCs. Contraction during a stressful event will dump large numbers of red cells and lymphocytes into the circulation, which can be reflected on the lab work, but it is not usually of any clinical significance. The elevations from these causes are relatively mild. However, there is a rare medical condition called *polycythemia* that can result in markedly elevated red blood cell counts. This is a serious condition that needs immediate medical attention. It often comes on slowly over time. The only thing you may notice is a loss of energy, excessive panting, and gum color that is bright (or "brick") red in color. The only way to determine if it is present is by performing blood work. Severely elevated red blood cell counts result in a sludging of the blood in the vessels, and serious blood clotting abnormalities can result.

There is also a condition called **hemorrhagic gastroenteritis** (HGE) which can result in massive quantities of fluid being dumped into the gastrointestinal (GI) tract. This fluid is pulled out of the circulation, so patients with **HGE** may experience **hemoconcentration**. Their PCV's can be in the 60-80% range. At this point, the blood is too thick to circulate properly, and a life-threatening clotting cascade may begin. HGE is a **true emergency** and is characterized by raspberry jam-like feces. IV fluids and aggressive therapy are necessary to stop the cycle.

NEWSFLASH

A PCV of less than 12% usually indicates the need for emergency blood transfusion.

A highly regenerative anemia is more often due to hemolysis rather than blood loss through injury or even parasites.

Non-regenerative anemias often have a worse prognosis.

Slow blood loss is better tolerated than rapid blood loss.

Section 2.2: White Blood Cells

Let's look at the other half of the CBC picture now, which measures the count and health of your pet's white blood cells. As well as the total white blood cell count, we're going to be talking here in more detail about the bottom section of the CBC tabulated results – this section:

Differential

Neutrophils	A type of white blood cells that forms a major defense in fighting infection
Bands	Immature neutrophils
Lymphocytes	A type of immune cell found in the blood and lymphatic tissue
Monocytes	A type of white blood cell that fights germs (viruses, bacteria, fungi, and protozoa) and eliminates infected cells
Eosinophils	A type of white blood cell most commonly activated when there is a parasitic infection, an allergic reaction, or cancer
Basophils	Least common white blood cell, important in early detection of some kinds of cancer and in some allergic responses

There are several distinct types of white blood cells within the total white blood cell count. If the overall count is increased, this usually indicates an infection or an inflammatory reaction. Sometimes the overall count is normal, but the individual cell lines are elevated or depressed.

White cells are known collectively as **leukocytes.** People who examine cells under microscopes divide white cells into two main types: **granulocytes** and **agranulocytes,** based on the presence or absence of tiny granules within the cell cytoplasm. Within these divisions, cells are further typed by function as well as their response to certain staining techniques. These distinctions aren't important to our discussion here except in how some people might refer to cells you know by a different name. What's important is what some of these cells respond to and what the significance of elevations in their numbers might mean.

Elevated WBC count

There are four main causes of an elevated white cell count, or **leukocytosis**:

- Inflammation or infection

- Stress/steroid therapy reaction, where there will be an elevated neutrophil count (no bands), decreased eosinophil count, decreased lymphocyte count, and an increased monocyte count. **NOTE**: A stress leukogram is a pattern, not a diagnosis!

- Exercise/excitement

- Leukemia

A **leukemoid reaction** is one in which the white cell numbers are greater than 50,000 – 100,000. This is a grave indicator of disease. If the source of the infection cannot be surgically removed (such as an infected uterus), then the prognosis for survival is poor.

Depressed WBC count

Panleukopenia is a general, across-the-board depression of ALL white cells and is usually indicative of bone marrow disease (which can also be indicated it the animal has a non-regenerative anemia, plus **thrombocytopenia**, which is a low platelet count).

Parvovirus can cause panleukopenia through bone marrow suppression. White cell counts under two thousand carry a grave-to-guarded prognosis in parvo puppies or kittens with feline distemper. Parvo in dogs developed in the 1970s when the cat distemper virus (also known as Panleukopenia, for the effects on the bone marrow) spontaneously mutated and began affecting dogs. It is NOT the same virus as canine distemper. In some severe parvo outbreaks, it is not unusual for unvaccinated kittens in the same shelter to develop symptoms if exposed.

Important definition: a word ending in "cytosis," or "philia" means elevation in number. "Penia" at the end of a word means a decrease in number.

Types of White Blood Cells

Neutrophils and Band Cells

Neutrophils are among the first line of defense. Think of them as foot soldiers in a vast war against infection. They can mobilize rapidly in large numbers when a breach in defenses has occurred, and infection threatens. Neutrophils move in a one-way direction from the bone marrow into the blood and tissues—foot soldiers aren't expected to survive the initial onslaught and return to the castle!

In general, an elevated white cell count (**leukocytosis**) is synonymous with an elevated neutrophil count (**neutrophilia**) because neutrophils make up the largest population of white cells. When you see pus in a wound, you're mostly seeing neutrophils, lymphocytes, and necrotic (dead) cellular material.

Neutrophils eat up infectious material, digest it, and die. Neutrophils remain in circulation approximately ten hours in normal circumstances and then drift into the respiratory, digestive, and urinary tracts as needed to clean up bacteria and debris.

Neutrophils are also called segmenters or "**segs**" because of the lobulated shape of the nucleus within the cell. Picture a snake that has swallowed several eggs—that is what the nucleus of a segmented neutrophil looks like. When an animal is battling infection, as the numbers of neutrophils become depleted, more immature neutrophils can be seen. Immature segs are called "**band**" cells because the "snake" in the middle is not segmented, but smooth like a banana.

If bands are noted in elevated numbers but the rest of the neutrophils are **normal to decreased** in number, this is called a "**left shift**." A left shift implies that the numbers of neutrophils are being deployed (and consumed) in greater numbers than they can be replaced. Picture those foot soldiers getting younger and younger as the war goes on and the "experienced" fighters have all been defeated.

The greater the number of band cells, the more serious the infection. If the infection continues to outstrip the ability of the body to replace the neutrophils, then the numbers will drop, resulting in a **neutropenia**. If a left shift is also present, this is considered a **degenerative** left shift. This carries a guarded-to-poor prognosis.

It is possible to have a neutropenia without the presence of band cells or a left shift, so a neutropenia on its own isn't necessarily an indication of a serious problem. The lab work must be viewed as a whole.

Neutrophils under heavy assault develop clear vacuoles ("empty places") within the cytoplasm. These are referred to as toxic changes or **toxic neutrophils**. Toxic changes can also be indicative of serious infection. The more toxic neutrophils you have, the more serious the infection.

Abnormally low levels of neutrophils (**neutropenia**) are uncommon and usually indicate excessive tissue consumption or primary bone marrow disease. Neutropenia due to excessive demand is likely to be supported by the increased presence of band cells. Certain types of gram-negative bacterial infections and rickettsial (tick-borne) diseases can lower neutrophil counts as well, usually by increased consumption.

Lymphocytes

Lymphocytes are the second line of defense. They are like the people stationed on the castle wall with buckets of boiling oil and flaming arrows. A high number of lymphocytes, especially in proportion to neutrophils, may indicate a chronic infection rather than an acute one. After an infection/invading host has been around for a while, the battle tends to shift away from neutrophils out in the field of battle, and the fighting gets close and dirty. Lymphocytes migrate in and out of lymphoid tissue (such as the spleen). Like defenders of the castle, they can move in and out of the "building." Think about those soldiers on the wall, popping in and out from behind the battlements.

- excessive lymphocyte numbers can also indicate a viral infection or immune-mediated problem, such as leukemia or hypothyroidism

- transient or temporary **lymphocytosis** (increased lymphocytes) can be seen in healthy cats that get excited during blood sampling or in all pets immediately after exercise or with the use of steroids.

- puppies normally have higher lymphocyte counts than adults.

Lymphocytes are divided into two types (**B cells** and **T cells**) according to function. They are responsible for creating antibodies and secreting enzymes that influence a wide number of cell types within the immune system. Most in-house lab machines are only going to report relative numbers of lymphocytes and not distinguish between the distinct types.

Reactive lymphocytes (supercharged, larger cells with dark cytoplasm) can occasionally be found in a normal blood smear but are sometimes seen in increased numbers in sick animals. They do not represent a specific disease but need to be differentiated by a trained cytologist from the cells of **lymphosarcoma** (cancer cells of the lymphoid tissue) or the cells seen in **acute lymphoblastic leukemia**. The take-home message here is reactive lymphocytes can be difficult to tell apart from more serious kinds of cells, and you need a trained eye to distinguish the two.

Decreased numbers of lymphocytes (**lymphopenia**) are seen in cases of long-term stress or steroid use. Lymphopenia is also expected in severe disease and certain diseases that result in the loss of lymph tissue, such as a protein-losing enteropathy in dogs (leaky bowels that cause impaired digestion of food and loss of cells into the gut).

Monocytes

Monocytes are baby **macrophages**. Monocytes circulate for a brief period before "growing up" and entering the tissues to become longer-acting macrophages. Macrophages are like knights in the castle defense system. They are large cells that remove pathogens, such as tissue debris, bacteria, fungi, cancer cells, and abnormal red cells. Macrophages also process foreign antigenic material and package it so that it can be handled by the lymphocytes. Another way of looking at it is that macrophages are at the end-stage of an inflammatory process.

Monocytosis is seen in cases of infections with lots of pus, tissue that is necrotic (dead or dying), malignant (aggressive cancers), hemolytic (the red cells are breaking up) or hemorrhagic (bleeding). If monocytosis is present in the absence of these things, a stress/steroid response is most likely.

The classic stress leukogram pattern is a mature **neutrophilia** (no bands) with a **lymphopenia, eosinopenia**, and **monocytosis**. If you have a monocytosis without these other characteristics, then look for possible chronic inflammation, such as bad skin or infected ears. A monocytosis alone, however, with no history or histopathology to back it up, is insufficient to prove chronic inflammation. Monocytopenia is not considered a significant finding in the dog or cat, as monocytes are usually in small numbers anyway and not evenly distributed in the bloodstream.

Eosinophils

Eosinophils, which normally make up less than 10% of the overall WBC, fight parasites and regulate the intensity of allergic reactions through the formation of antibodies. They are attracted to inflamed tissues by the release of certain chemical markers released by the damaged cells. Imagine that parts of the castle have caught on fire: the eosinophils rush to that area to stomp the fire out.

For a strong eosinophil response to parasites, the parasite must invade the tissues. Parasites that migrate through tissue (such as heartworms or lung flukes) may create a big enough response that increase eosinophil counts in the bloodstream. Fleas often trigger allergic reactions to their saliva, so a flea infestation may also trigger an eosinophilia. Viral, bacterial, and fungal infections as well as food allergies can be another source of elevated eosinophils.

Basophils

Basophils are white cells that are present in extremely low numbers in the general circulation. Elevations are triggered by the same conditions that cause eosinophilia; they can also be elevated when **lipemia** occurs in the blood (free circulation of fat in the bloodstream.) Many in-house chemistry machines do not recognize basophils individually, so if they are identified at all, it is by microscopic examination of a blood smear by a trained technician. They are easy to misidentify and do not often play a significant role in most inflammatory reactions.

Leukemia

Leukemia is a condition characterized by a **grossly elevated leukocyte count** or when the white cells appear abnormal (back to that need for someone to visualize the cell morphology again). Final diagnosis is made on bone marrow evaluation (bone marrow is the originating source of all white cells) by a trained pathologist. Prognosis is poor in cases of true leukemia, but some forms may respond to surgery or chemotherapy. There are many different forms of leukemia, and the classifications change frequently, so we won't discuss it in detail here. Suffice to say, it is a serious medical condition, typically best treated by a specialist.

Feline leukemia is a virus that causes several different syndromes, one of which is outright leukemia in cats. To date, the prognosis for cats with feline leukemia is poor with 97% of cats testing positive succumbing to one of the various syndromes within three years of testing positive. Because this is a contagious disease spread by biting, fighting, and mating, it is recommended that cats with FeLV be isolated from negative status cats. Because their immune systems are compromised, illness in a FeLV + cat needs to be treated more aggressively than in a seronegative cat. Cats that have access to the outdoors and can come into contact with other cats in the community should be tested and vaccinated against Feline Leukemia.

Acute Inflammation, Allergic Reactions, and Mast Cells

Mast cells are filled with reactive (primarily histamine) granules that they release in acute inflammatory disorders and allergic reactions. **Anaphylaxis**, a state where the body goes into acute shock due to an allergic reaction, is the result of large numbers of mast cells degranulating at the same time.

Mast cells are not identified on a blood smear unless **mast cell neoplasia** (cancer) occurs and sometimes not even then. They are most readily identified by an examination of a "buffy coat smear," a microscopic examination of the white cell layer that forms on top of the packed red cells in a hematocrit tube. This layer might be examined if a mast cell tumor has been diagnosed and your vet is looking for evidence of **metastasis** (spreading to distant parts of the body), but this procedure is no longer considered to be a valid way to assess prognosis for survivability with mast cell cancer. Mast cells are often readily identified in needle aspirates of mast cell tumors.

NEWSFLASH

Large numbers of band cells with a normal to decreased neutrophil count are BAD.

White cell counts of 50,000 - 100,000 are BAD (unless infection can be removed.)

If eosinophils are up, look for parasites or allergies.

A "stress leukogram" describes a specific white cell pattern; it is not a diagnosis.

More on Ralphie's case study: Parvovirus

Remember Ralphie's CBC? Well, let's look at it again:

Test Requested	Results	Reference Range	Units
Hemoglobin	9.1 (**LOW**)	12.1-20.3	g/dl
Hematocrit	15 (**LOW**)	33-45%	
WBC	4.4	4-15.5	$10^3/\mu l$
RBC	3.2 (**LOW**)	4.8-9.3	
Platelet count	180	170-400	
Platelet estimate	adequate	Adequate	
Reticulocytes	3 % (elevated)		

Differential	Absolute	%	Range
Neutrophils	2772	63	2060-10600
Bands	0	0	0-300
Lymphocytes	388	7	690-4500
Eosinophils	800 ***	18 (**H**)	0-1200
Basophils	0	0	0-150

This time we are going to concentrate on the part of the CBC that begins under the "differential." Here are all our white blood cell friends that we just talked about—the neutrophils, the lymphocytes...etc. Note in this example that there are no bands (hooray!), and that even though the overall number of eosinophils is within normal limits, the relative percentage of eosinophils is elevated. This is entirely consistent with Ralphie being heavily infested with fleas and worms thus becoming anemic as a result. Don't get stressed if the readout doesn't exactly match what you may be given on your own dog. Remember, different labs report information differently.

Suppose Ralphie developed parvovirus, and we took just the differential numbers into consideration here. If Ralphie had a total WBC of 2200 (which is significantly decreased), his differential might look something like this:

Differential	Absolute	%	
Neutrophils	1500	68	2060-10600
Bands	400	18	0-300
Lymphocytes	90	4	690-4500
Monocytes	10	0.45	0-840
Eosinophils	0	0	0-1200
Basophils	0	0	0-150

Okay, I don't know about you right now, but I am getting really worried about Ralphie's ability to survive this outbreak of parvovirus. First, ALL Ralphie's white cell numbers are depressed across the board—this is because among other things, parvo causes **panleukopenia,** which is a suppression of white cell production at the level of the bone marrow. Markedly low white cell counts decrease the chances for survival of this disease because the body doesn't have anything with which to fight off infection.

Secondly, Ralphie's elevated band count indicates he has a **left shift;** his overworked bone marrow is trying to send out babies to do a soldier's job. We must treat Ralphie aggressively with IV fluids (because he is pouring out great volumes of fluids and electrolytes in his vomit and diarrhea) as well as antibiotics in hopes of fending off secondary **sepsis** (bacterial infection in the blood) from his suppressed immune system. Since the damaged gastrointestinal surface can weep bacteria in large numbers into the bloodstream, secondary bacterial infections can be life-threatening. The antibiotics will not treat the parvo virus itself.

Parvo is a nasty, ugly disease that came out of nowhere in the 1970's when it mutated from a common cat virus—feline distemper—which we mentioned before. In addition to the effect that it has on the white cell counts and fluid losses, it can directly attack the muscles of the heart and cause sudden myocardial death in a puppy that appears to be recovering well. Sections of bowel can stop moving properly (**ileus**) and parts of the still-moving bowels can telescope over the dead-in-the-water bowels, resulting in an intestinal impaction or **intussusception** that can only be untangled (or removed) surgically. Puppies that receive aggressive fluid therapy and medical support stand the best chance of surviving parvo, but we still lose puppies every year to this terrible disease. Some of the newer flu medications have been shown to shorten the severity and length of illness if started early in the course of infection, so be sure to discuss these treatment options with your veterinarian if necessary. Tamiflu does not target the parvo virus directly but has effects on neuraminidase, which is an important enzyme used by gut bacteria to by-pass the protective barriers of the gut walls. As such, it may help prevent sepsis, though its use in parvo puppies is still considered controversial.

More on Muffy

Remember Muffy? Well, instead of her having autoimmune hemolytic anemia, we'll make her an intact (unspayed) female dog that was in heat four or five weeks ago and is now vomiting, refusing to eat, and drinking lots of water.

Test	Results		
WBC	75 $10^3/\mu l$		
Differential	**absolute**	**%**	**Range**
Neutrophils	60,000	80	2060-10600
Bands	400	0.5	0-300
Lymphocytes	7,000	9.3	690-4500
Monocytes	7,600	10	0-840
Eosinophils	0	0	0-1200
Basophils	0	0	0-150

Yikes! Muffy's WBC is really elevated, and it is largely made up of neutrophils. Even though the band numbers are the same as Ralphie's in the last example, you can see that because the overall neutrophil numbers are elevated, the total percentage of WBCs that are bands is lower than in Ralphie's case, so this is NOT a left shift. However, WBC numbers of this magnitude in a dog with this history and these clinical signs means you should be looking for a serious infection. In Muffy's case, radiographs (x-rays to you and me) or abdominal ultrasound should be performed to rule out a uterine infection (**pyometra**).

Section 2.3: Platelets

Platelets (**thrombocytes**) are part of the blood clotting mechanism, and dysfunction of the platelets is the most common cause of bleeding problems. Like red cells and white cells, platelets are also produced by the bone marrow. They are actually pieces of large cells called megakaryocytes, which break off and circulate in the bloodstream to help form clots and slow down bleeding. Decreased platelet production can be an indication of bone marrow disease.

Platelet count

When evaluating the platelet count, we must be sure that excessive clotting hasn't occurred during the collection procedure, as this will give us a falsely decreased estimate of platelets numbers. In certain diseases, such as Von Willebrand syndrome, it's possible for the platelet numbers to be adequate, but because the platelets themselves don't function properly, clotting is still an issue. Certain **platelet function** tests may be needed to determine the difference between inadequate numbers verses a platelet dysfunction disorder.

Autoimmune disorders

Platelets, like red blood cells, are vulnerable to increased destruction either through autoimmune mechanisms or through excessive consumption. Many different drug therapies (including some common antibiotics) as well as some vaccines have been implicated in triggering an autoimmune destruction cascade in some patients. In **autoimmune thrombocytopenia (AIT)**, a foreign protein called a **hapten** attaches to the platelet, causing the body to think it is an intruder. Think of the platelets as wearing little hats: the body doesn't recognize this "stranger" and shoots it down.

While AIT is a severe immune disorder, most pets respond to medication. However, sometimes pets with AIT have another underlying problem causing the thrombocytopenia. The prognosis is more guarded in those cases, as many of those animals tend not to respond to treatment.

When platelet numbers fall to the 35,000-50,000 range, spontaneous bleeding (such as nosebleeds or bruising under the skin) may occur. Such marked thrombocytopenia is usually associated with an autoimmune problem. Less severe thrombocytopenia can be seen from other causes, such as tick-borne diseases like Lyme disease.

Giant platelets

Giant platelets can sometimes be seen in conditions when the counts are low due to excessive destruction of platelets. This may also be an inherited condition (versus a clinical one) in Cavalier King Charles Spaniels (CKCS). This breed commonly exhibits the presence of **macrothrombocytopenia,** which is a combination of giant platelets and low platelet numbers. Platelet counts in these dogs can be strikingly low (ranging from 30-90,000) but unlike other breeds of dogs, CKCS rarely have signs of bleeding.

Some diagnostic labs recommend performing a manual platelet count on this breed as automated counters can't accurately identify the giant platelets and will often misidentify them as red blood cells.

Clotting

While it is not a routine part of the CBC, this might be a good place to talk about clotting profiles. These specialized tests are run when we suspect there is a problem with normal coagulation, either due to an abnormality with the platelets because of something that is interfering with the clotting mechanism, or because of primary **hemophilia** (a bleeding disorder that makes even a tiny cut potentially life-threatening).

Coagulation factors in the blood are divided into pathways. The different branches are called the Intrinsic, Extrinsic, and Common pathways. This only becomes important when we look at the results of the various tests to measure coagulation function. The information is then used to narrow down the source of the abnormality.

Tests for abnormal **prothrombin** times (**PT**) measure how long the blood takes to clot. The most common cause of prolonged PT, where the blood is taking too long to clot, is exposure to rat poisons which cause problems with Vitamin K-related "factors," such as Factor VII. In fact, bleeding problems because of rat poison will show up there first. The important thing to remember is that if you suspect rat poison, it won't hurt for the vet to start your pet on Vitamin K until the blood work results come back, and it could potentially save your pet's life. We're talking about a medical prescription of Vitamin K here, which is in excess of what might be in a commercial dog food.

PT is often run as part of a coagulation profile along with **Activated Partial Prothrombin Time (APPT)**, which screens for other coagulation deficiencies, such as hemophilia. Since this gets very complicated, more in-depth discussion of bleeding disorders is beyond the scope of this text.

Additional tests to evaluate platelet function might include **buccal mucosa bleeding time (BMBT)**. A spring-loaded device is used to create a standardized slice on the surface of the lip of your pet. The time it takes for a clot to form should be around 3 minutes—but I'll be honest, I can't recall the last time I saw one of these used in a clinical setting, despite the fact that is a sensitive and accurate test. No one likes intentionally cutting a patient to see how long it takes for bleeding to stop!

NEWSFLASH

Severely decreased platelet counts are almost always immune-mediated.

A dog can have normal platelet numbers but can still have a clotting disorder.

The CBC: Conclusion

This has been a lot to take in on the CBC, I know. But hopefully, you now have a better understanding of the CBC, enough so you can ask your vet questions and understand the answers.

Section 3: The Chemistry Profile

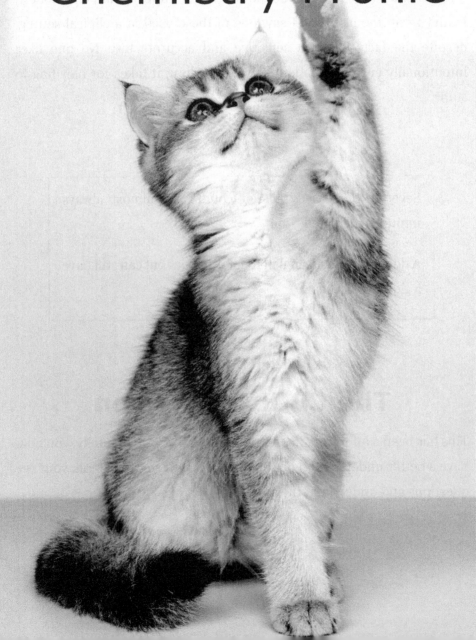

The Chemistry Profile

The chemistry ("chem") profile measures anywhere from 6-15 different enzymes, minerals, and electrolytes that are produced by various organs and circulate in the bloodstream. It is a vital step in the analysis of metabolic function in your pet.

The degree to which a complete profile should be performed depends on why you need to know. Many labs and in-house chemistry machines offer abbreviated testing as a part of a wellness check or pre-anesthetic screening. But a geriatric or sick pet, any animal that is "not doing right," an animal with chronic weight loss, or an animal with changes in water consumption and/or urine output should have a more complete profile. Ideally, your pet should be fasted before testing because a recent meal can affect some values, but fasting is not always possible or desirable.

The profile can be divided into distinct categories based on what organ systems can be evaluated through the measurement of certain enzymes. In general:

- **Kidneys**: BUN, creatinine

- **Liver**: ALT, ALKP, bilirubin

- **Pancreas:** amylase, lipase, blood glucose

- **Minerals**: Calcium (Ca+), Phosphorus (Phos)

- **Electrolytes**: Sodium (Na+), Potassium (K+), Chloride (Cl-)

As always, the normal ranges for these values can vary depending on the equipment used, so results must be compared to the normal ranges provided by the laboratory that performed the lab work. Also, be aware that hospitals that use human laboratories may use different names for some of the liver enzymes or may include enzymes that are not routinely evaluated in pet medicine.

The ranges may also be slightly different based on the species in question. Lab machines calibrated for animals will frequently take the species into consideration when evaluating the test results.

Section 3.1: The Kidney Values

Blood urea nitrogen (BUN)

BUN is not technically a kidney (**renal**) enzyme, but it is more strongly associated with kidney function than other organs. BUN is a waste product from the liver, arising from the breakdown of protein in the diet, and is filtered out of the body by the kidneys. BUN can be affected by other factors so can't be relied on solely as a determination of kidney function. It must *always* be evaluated in relation to creatinine levels and urine specific gravity.

- **BUN: normal (6-24 mg/dl)**

Elevated BUN Levels

If there is significant kidney dysfunction, the BUN levels will rise because the kidneys are no longer filtering it properly, creating a condition known as **azotemia**.

Think of the bloodstream as a fast-running creek. Now picture this creek flowing into a reservoir that has a pump house with a filter at the head of the pond. The pump house represents the kidneys, and the reservoir represents the bladder. On the other end of the reservoir is a sluice that periodically opens and allows the reservoir to drain (the urinary sphincter that opens to allow urination).

The kidney is much more complicated than a simple filter but go with me here. On a normal day with a working filter, toxic levels of BUN are actively pumped and filtered out of the creek into the reservoir to be removed from the system. But if the pump/filter is bad, the levels of BUN begin to back up in the creek until the creek is so tainted, the water becomes poisonous, and fish begin to die. This is what happens when the kidneys are unable to do their job in filtering BUN from the bloodstream.

What if less water is coming through the filter in the first place? Well, just like the relative amount of "gravel" in the fish tank seems higher when there is less water, less water in the system will "raise" BUN levels. This is how dehydration can make BUN levels appear elevated.

What if the sluice doesn't open properly? Well, eventually the reservoir would back up through the filter and into the bloodstream, also resulting in elevated BUN levels. This would be the case if a stone (or urinary crystals in a male cat) became lodged in the urethra and prevented the voiding of urine—a life-threatening emergency. In this case, removal of the obstruction should allow the BUN should go back to normal. Only in the case of a true filter problem would you be dealing with real kidney dysfunction.

If the **creatinine** levels are normal, mild to moderate elevations of BUN could be due to a recent canned or raw meat meal. Extra protein in the diet (including blood proteins from chronic gastrointestinal bleeding), dehydration, massive muscle trauma, or extreme muscle wasting (typical of certain cancers as well as cardiac and kidney diseases) also result in mild-moderate BUN elevations in the face of normal creatinine levels. This is important because the creatinine levels are much more closely tied into kidney function than the BUN levels are. So, if the BUN is elevated, but the creatinine levels are normal, you need to look at other disease processes and disorders besides kidney failure.

If the **urine specific gravity** (a measurement of the kidney's ability to concentrate urine—there's more detail on this subject under the description of the urinalysis later) indicates a normal ability to concentrate urine, then the BUN elevations are pre-renal ("in front of the kidneys") in source. So, an elevated BUN with normal creatinine levels in a well-hydrated dog can be an indicator of bleeding into the GI tract. The stool should be examined for signs of blood (either fresh blood or black, tarry **melena,** which is digested blood), and your dog should be screened for intestinal parasites.

If the creatinine is **also** significantly elevated, then the BUN elevations are renal (kidney) in source – they aren't filtering properly. An exception would be the post-renal urinary obstruction. In which case, the animal would be unable to urinate. If the animal is capable of voiding urine and that urine is very dilute (low urine specific gravity), and both the BUN and creatinine are elevated, think kidney failure. Other causes of decreased filtration would be systemic shock or poor cardiac output, which would alter filtration rate because of a decrease in volume of fluid passing through it.

Decreased BUN Levels

Causes include decreased protein intake, chronic liver insufficiency (resulting in decreased production), over-hydration due to excessive fluid therapy or water consumption (as in diabetes or Cushing's disease), which dilutes the percentage of BUN circulating at a given time. But because the BUN is a by-product of the liver, a persistently decreased BUN indicates a need for further liver function tests.

To complicate matters, significant kidney damage must occur before you'll see elevations in BUN and creatine together. As much as 77% of kidney function must be compromised before these values will change. Idexx Laboratories now has a screening test called SDMA which can detect kidney compromise at a much earlier level, allowing for intervention at an earlier stage. SDMA stands for symmetric dimethylarginine (SDMA). This is an amino acid that is produced at a constant rate as a result of the breakdown of proteins by most of the cells. Because it is usually filtered out of the body by the kidneys, it can be used as a measurement of kidney function. Staging renal disease allows veterinarians to make dietary and medical recommendations based on the degree of compromise.

Creatinine

Creatinine (CREAT) is produced in small quantities in the body. There is a direct correlation between creatinine levels and the rate of kidney filtration.

- **Creatinine: normal (0.4-1.5 mg/dl)**

Elevated Creatinine Levels

Elevation of creatinine levels almost always indicates decreased kidney filtration rate – the kidneys just aren't filtering waste properly. The body tolerates only a very narrow normal range of creatinine levels, so even small elevations can be clinically significant. If other causes of decreased filtration are not obviously present (such as shock or heart failure), then the decreased filtration is due to poor kidney function.

There are few non-renal factors that can influence creatinine levels. The same factors that can affect filtration rate (such as shock...etc.) can cause false elevations in creatinine, but as the underlying condition is corrected, the levels will also self-correct. Sometimes, though, other issues can alter levels. If free fat is floating in the bloodstream (blood is **lipemic**), or if the patient is taking vitamin C and/or a wide variety of medications or antibiotics, creatinine "lookalikes" can occur which are misread by some chemistry machines as creatinine itself. If the BUN is normal and your pet is taking supplements or medication, consult with your veterinarian about discontinuing the supplemented product for two weeks and repeat the creatinine levels to see if they are truly elevated or not.

High BUN and creatinine together indicate primary kidney dysfunction. If the phosphorous levels are also high and the red blood count is low (indicating possible decreased erythropoietin production by the kidneys), the problem is chronic **kidney failure**, especially if there is significant weight loss as well. Severe, chronic elevations carry a poor-guarded prognosis in the older animal.

Decreased Creatinine Levels

It's not very common, but creatinine levels can be decreased in cases of significant muscle loss (such as cancer **cachexia** where the body's metabolic needs are so high that the body itself is breaking down), or when increased cardiac output or pregnancy results in an increased kidney filtration rate.

Renal failure: urine specific gravity testing

Evaluation of the **urine specific gravity** can help determine if the kidney retains any concentrating ability. A common misconception is that excessive urination is an indicator of normally functioning kidneys. When I mention the possibility of kidney failure, many clients are in disbelief because their pets are urinating excessively—how could the kidneys have failed? The reason behind this that as the kidneys are starting to fail, the "filter" may not be retaining any water for the body's needs. Thus, as fast as their pet drinks water, it goes out the other end. If the kidney (through an active filtration pump mechanism) is not able to retain enough water for the body's uses, dehydration will result as water, in the form of dilute urine, leaves the body faster than it can be replaced.

A healthy pump system will concentrate the urine to its maximum capacity, even in the face of outgoing losses (such as vomiting) or decreased input (such as lack of access to water). An animal with healthy kidneys can still dehydrate in this type of situation if it lasts long enough, but the urine specific gravity will be maximally concentrated. Animals in kidney failure will become progressively more dehydrated even in the presence of free-choice water because they cannot concentrate their urine normally, and the urine specific gravity will reflect this.

Acute renal failure (sudden onset due to a toxic/infectious agent) may sometimes have a better prognosis with aggressive therapy if the source of the damage can be identified and eliminated. In general, dogs are not as tolerant of significant kidney disease compared to some other species and are more difficult to manage long term. Cats can often survive for years with not-so-great kidneys, whereas they do not seem to tolerate diseases of the lungs as well as dogs. Every species has its strengths and weaknesses when it comes to survival.

Antech Diagnostic Laboratories examined clinical blood test parameters on dogs being fed different types of raw diets verses dry kibble and determined the following: dogs eating a raw diet have a higher average

BUN than dogs eating dry kibble (due to the greater protein content of most raw diets). Dogs eating specifically the Volhard NDF diet also had greater average creatinine values. Healthy dogs maintained a higher but still normal range on these tests. This has led Antech to consider further study as to whether lab parameters need to factor in diet when calculating normal ranges for these tests. It may also be a factor to consider when the dog in question does not have healthy kidney function and we are looking to reduce those blood values.

NEWSFLASH

High BUN and creatinine together indicate kidney dysfunction

High phosphorus levels plus low RBC levels suggests chronic kidney failure

Chronic weight loss plus kidney failure carries a guarded prognosis

Risk Factors for Kidney Disease

Breed

Some breeds of dogs and cats have a higher incidence rate of kidney disease than others. There can be many causes for this, including a hereditary component. So, you may want to perform lab work on these dogs more often or run additional screening tests that can detect problems before it is reflected in the bloodwork (more tests are discussed under the urinalysis section). We use the term **familial nephropathies (disorders of the kidneys)** to describe these syndromes when it is not always clear how the problem is inherited, but it is present in higher-than-normal numbers within certain breeds. The rate of progression of disease depends on the breed and the type of nephropathy.

Familial nephropathies in dogs and cats

Dogs

Renal Dysplasia

- o Lhasa Apso
- o Shih Tzu
- o Standard Poodle
- o Soft-Coated Wheaten Terrier
- o Chow Chow
- o Alaskan Malamute
- o Miniature Schnauzer
- o Dutch Kooiker (Dutch Decoy) Dog

Primary glomerulopathies

- o Samoyed and Navasota (X-linked-passes through the female line)
- o English Cocker Spaniel (autosomal recessive-both parents must pass on the abnormal gene)
- o Bull Terrier (autosomal dominant)
- o Dalmatian (autosomal dominant)
- o Doberman Pinscher
- o Bullmastiff
- o Newfoundland

- o   Rottweiler
- o   Pembroke Welsh Corgi
- o   Beagle

Polycystic kidney disease

- o   Bull Terrier (autosomal dominant)
- o   Carin Terrier and West Highland White Terrier (autosomal recessive)

Amyloidosis

- o   Shar Pei
- o   English Foxhound
- o   Beagle

Immune-mediated glomerulonephritis

- o   Soft-Coated Wheaton Terrier
- o   Bernese Mountain Dog (autosomal recessive, suspected)
- o   Brittany Spaniel (autosomal recessive)

Miscellaneous

- o   Basenji - Fanconi syndrome
- o   German Shepherd - multifocal cystadenocarcinoma (autosomal dominant)
- o   Pembroke Welsh Corgi – telangiectasia

Cats

Polycystic kidney disease

- o   Persian (autosomal dominant)

Amyloidosis

- o   Abyssinian (autosomal dominant with incomplete penetrance, suspected)
- o   Siamese and Oriental

The bottom line is that if you have a purebred pet, you'll need to do your research to learn what kinds of hereditary problems they might have and plan to manage them. Mixed breed dogs are subject to the problems of their predominant breeds, so if your dog is identifiably part Lhasa or part Chow, you can think about what kinds of problems might be inherited.

The rate of progression of these familial nephropathies varies widely with the breed and type of nephritis seen. Please be aware that your veterinarian may not be familiar with all the variations and risk factors in your purebred dog. Your vet is going to be aware of the tendency of cocker spaniels to get autoimmune hemolytic anemia because it is a frequent problem in a popular breed. If you have a less common breed of dog (for example, a Soft-coated Wheaten or a Bull Terrier), then it is up to you as an informed caretaker to be aware of the potential genetic tendencies of that breed.

Today it is possible to get DNA testing done on your dog. Not only is it fun to see what the genetic makeup of your dog might be, but many of these tests also screen for a host of genetic diseases, including the **multidrug resistance gene (MDR1)**, which can affect how your dog processes a wide variety of medications.

Infections

Chronic urinary tract infections can lead to **pyelonephritis** (a kidney infection):

- A common example of this would be the dog with a disc injury that is now incapable of completely emptying the bladder. Urine pooling in the bladder will eventually grow bacteria.

- A dog with a neurologic bladder is very prone to urinary tract infections and may well have some degree of infection all the time. It is possible for such an infection to move backwards up the ureters and infect the kidneys.

- Diabetic animals are also prone to kidney infections because of the intermittent presence of excess sugar in the urine.

- Some animals are prone to recurrent urinary tract infections (UTIs) because of the presence of stones or some anatomical changes.

- As female dogs age, many begin leaking urine because of a weak urinary sphincter. A sphincter that allows urine to leak out also can allow bacteria to sneak in.

Some blood-borne infections can result in pyelonephritis because within the kidneys is a large blood supply associated with them as part of their duty as a filtration system. The kidneys are therefore highly susceptible to **septicemia** (an infection in the blood) because they are filtering blood to remove waste, and the infection can take hold in the kidneys themselves, damaging the **nephrons** (the individual units of kidney filtration). Such damage is often permanent, as the body doesn't have the ability to make new nephrons (which is why, in humans, kidney transplants are sometimes the only remedy to resolve renal failure). However, kidney function *can* improve and even return to normal after an infection because there are so many nephrons present and some compensation occurs. Nephron death occurs as a normal part of aging, and kidney function declines as we get older, so having fewer nephrons following an infection will put your dog at a disadvantage when aging changes occur.

One infectious disease we vaccinate dogs against is called **leptospirosis,** spread in the urine of deer, cattle, mice, and racoons. Leptospirosis can result in acute renal failure (this is the most common presenting clinical sign). With the correct diagnosis and aggressive treatment with antibiotics and fluids, Lepto has an 80% survival rate but can cause permanent liver and kidney damage. It is also a **zoonotic** disease, meaning it can be spread to humans.

Tick-borne diseases such as Lyme have become increasingly common in parts of the U.S. and can also cause permanent kidney damage.

Drug Therapy/Toxic Exposure

A wide selection of medication can result in kidney damage, some of the most common falling into the classes of antimicrobials (especially aminoglycoside antibiotics) and certain antifungal medications (amphotericin B). These medications are usually chosen with great care and consideration for the risk–benefit ratio for a particular animal.

Also in this category are many non-steroidal anti-inflammatories (including aspirin and ibuprofen) and many chemotherapeutic agents (such as cisplatin and methotrexate). Use of these medications may require extra monitoring of kidney function. Dogs and cats are particularly sensitive to the side effects of non-steroidal anti-inflammatories (NSAIDs), and even therapeutic doses can result in liver and kidney damage in some cases.

One of the most common causes of toxic renal failure is ingestion of ibuprofen. The lethal dose of ibuprofen is quite small on a milligram-per-kilogram basis and the consumption of a bottle of headache pills can prove fatal. **Never give ibuprofen or Tylenol to your pets!** One extra-strength Tylenol can kill your cat. In fact, you should never give any human over-the-counter medication to your pets, as many products contain ingredients that your pet cannot safely consume.

While you may find recommendations online for "safe" doses of aspirin for your dog, dogs are particularly susceptible to the ulcer-causing effects of aspirin, and it should never be given long-term to your pet. There is no difference between human aspirin and "dog" aspirin when it comes to active ingredients. Calling something "dog" aspirin doesn't make it safer for your dog to take.

Antifreeze ingestion is one of the most common causes of toxic-induced renal failure. Antifreeze (ethylene glycol) is converted into formaldehyde in the body by an enzyme called alcohol dehydrogenase. This ingestion causes crystals to form in the urine and within the kidneys, resulting in severe damage. In the initial stages of antifreeze poisoning (as this chemical reaction is taking place), your dog might exhibit "drunk-like" behavior. If caught early enough, your vet can attempt to tie up all the available enzymes by flooding the body with a grain alcohol solution (or chemical equivalent) in an IV drip. Your vet must keep your dog on the verge of alcohol poisoning to do this! The alcohol competes for the enzyme and prevents the chemical reaction from taking place in your dog's body.

There are some additional, newer treatments that can help improve the prognosis in the case of antifreeze ingestion, but all too often antifreeze proves to be fatal. Antifreeze is sweet, and animals tend to lick puddles found on the ground. Even a small amount can prove deadly, and many times, the pet owner didn't even see their pet consume it. Some of the newer antifreeze products have had a bitter additive added. I can't think why they all don't have this treatment done.

Soft-moist foods (those foods that resemble fake meat bits or hamburger) usually contain propylene glycol as an additive. Propylene glycol is chemically related to ethylene glycol, which is the active ingredient in antifreeze. **Dogs fed foods containing propylene glycol may cross-react and test falsely positive on an antifreeze test.** This is valuable information for your veterinarian to have if the question of antifreeze exposure comes up. Propylene glycol can cause a Heinz body anemia (a condition where red blood cells are destroyed) when fed to cats. This is when the food additive causes clumps of damaged hemoglobin inside the red cells, which then alters the flexibility of the cells. Inflexible red blood cells fracture when passing through small capillaries, instead of adapting to the shape of the blood vessels. I recommend avoiding feeding your pet food listing propylene glycol. There are times it has medical uses (like raising blood sugar in ewes with pregnancy toxemia), but it should never be fed on a regular basis.

Be sure to notify your vet if your pet consumes these types of foods in the advent of a potential antifreeze scare. Better yet, don't feed this type of food!

Another danger to your pet is a new sugar substitute called xylitol. Six pieces of xylitol-flavored gum can kill a large dog, causing liver failure. Don't use it in your baking or leave products containing it where your pet can get at it. Worse, many products such as peanut butter, yogurt, and certain human medications might contain xylitol as a flavoring. Read your labels before sharing that spoon of yogurt with your pet!

Cats are particularly sensitive to all NSAIDs, which makes treating them for pain challenging. There are very few pain medications labeled for use in cats in the US, and all of them have the potential for severe side effects.

You should have a discussion with your vet any time such medications are prescribed as to the risk–benefit ratio.

Age

As our pets get older, the risk of chronic renal failure increases. Kidney function decreases due to nephrons dying off (attrition) at a time when your dog may be taking multiple medications that can also affect kidney function. Medication may need to be altered accordingly and increased monitoring is recommended.

Ischemia

This is a condition where blood supply is severely altered, either due to trauma resulting in shock or profound blood loss, or heart problems resulting in decreased output. Anesthesia without IV fluid support can result in ischemia to weakened kidneys. Another cause is that many of the older non-steroidal anti-inflammatories (NSAIDs) inhibit prostaglandins, which are the mediators of pain and inflammation. The only problem is there are good prostaglandins as well that promote healthy perfusion of the kidneys and form a protective lining in the stomach against ulcers.

Some of the newer NSAIDs by-pass the "good" prostaglandins and only work on the "bad" ones, which can help protect both the kidneys and the stomach against issues.

Diabetes Mellitus (DM)

In people, advanced cases of DM cause damage to the network of tiny blood vessels in the kidneys. This is not seen as often in dogs because of their shorter life span (they do not typically live with diabetes for greater than 20 years) but is a potential complication of your dog's DM is uncontrolled. It may be hard for you to notice DM at first because both diabetic dogs and dogs with renal problems drink more water and urinate more frequently. A well-controlled diabetic dog should not be consuming excessive amounts of water, however. A urinalysis will identify loss of urine-concentrating ability as well as increased protein levels in the urine. If urine glucose is also present, then the DM is not well-controlled either.

Case Study: Barker

Barker is a 14-year-old cocker spaniel. He has been gradually losing weight over the last six months and has lost a total of four pounds since his last visit. He came to the clinic because he is urinating in the house and has begun to vomit.

Barker's bloodwork: on CBC shows PCV 24% (L) with no reticulocytes, WBC within normal limits. His chemistry profile results are:

Test	Results	Reference Range	Units
Albumin (ALB)	3.08	2.7-4.4	g/dl
Alkaline phosphatase (ALKP)	116	5-131	U/L

Test	Results	Reference Range	Units
Alanine transferase (ALT)	33	12-118	U/L
Amylase (AMYL)	553	500-1500	U/L
Blood Urea Nitrogen (BUN)	100 (H)	6-25	mg/dl
Calcium (Ca)	9.92	8.9-11.4	mg/dl
Cholesterol (CHOL)	292.2	92-324	mg/dl
Creatinine (CREA)	4 (H)	0.5-1.8	mg/dl
Glucose (GLU)	103.4	70-138	mg/dl
Phosphorus (PHOS)	16 (H)	2.5-6.0	mg/dl
Total bilirubin (TBILI)	0.26	0.00-0.90	mg/dl
Total Protein (TP)	6.37	5.2-8.2	g/dl

Test	Results	Reference Range	Units
Globulins (GLOB)	3.28	2.5-4.5	g/dl

The chemistry values of note have an H for High or an L for Low.

The presence of elevated BUN plus creatinine indicates a primary kidney problem. The increased phosphorous puts Barker at risk for developing **pseudohypoparathyroidism syndrome** (the bones become "rubbery" due to improper mineral balance). The decreased red blood cell count and the non-regenerative anemia (no reticulocytes, or "baby" red blood cells to the rescue) in addition to the weight loss indicates a chronic rather than an acute onset of illness. The vomiting is due to the toxic effect of the BUN on the gastrointestinal system and ulceration may be present. If significant GI ulceration is present, Barker could also have **melena** (black, tarry-looking stools). More than likely, Barker's urine specific gravity (more on this later) would be very dilute (around 1.010). The presumptive diagnosis in this case would be chronic renal failure.

The severity of the clinical signs plus the evidence of **chronic renal failure** creates a guarded prognosis for Barker.

Section 3.2: The Liver Values

There are many liver enzymes. Older practitioners or clinics that use human laboratories may refer to these enzymes by other names and include those that may not have as much significance in the dog and cat as they do in human medicine. For example, GGT is a liver enzyme that is often used to monitor relapse of alcoholism in people but has less practical purpose in vet medicine! For clarity's sake, let's limit our discussion to the most reviewed liver enzymes and their clinical significance.

ALT

ALT (alanine transferase) is an enzyme that indicates damage to the liver cells themselves (hepatocellular damage)—it comes from **inside** leaky liver cells. It doesn't hang around in the body very long (it has a short half-life of 1-2 days), so persistent elevations indicate **ongoing** liver cell damage. Because it is very specific to the liver cells, it is preferentially measured over some other, similar enzymes that are not as specific.

- **ALT (alanine transferase): Normals vary with lab**

Unfortunately, even though elevations indicate liver damage is occurring, measurement of this enzyme can't pinpoint the causes of damage. For example, an increased ALT can be due to any drug causing increased hepatocellular permeability (the cell's "leakiness"). There are a wide variety of medications that can do this, even medications that are considered safe in most patients. To make matters more confusing, significant elevations do not directly correlate with the *amount* of liver damage.

ALT levels are frequently elevated in cats with **hyperthyroidism**. These cats are under an extreme amount of physical stress, due to the catabolic energy drain the thyroid disease causes as well as the strain on the heart and other organs. These values will usually return to normal when the thyroid levels are controlled. If someone brings me a skinny, senior cat, and I discover elevated ALT levels on the lab work, you can bet I'm going to order a thyroid test if I haven't already done so!

Because the liver is the "trash can" of the body, responsible for filtering out many toxic, viral, and bacterial agents, often a liver biopsy is needed to determine the underlying cause of persistent ALT elevations. Unfortunately, many of the animals that need a liver biopsy the most are also the patients at elevated risk for anesthesia. A biopsy is something that needs to be decided on an individual basis between you and your veterinarian. What's more, since the liver is also responsible for producing many of the blood clotting "factors," **a clotting profile is recommended before any liver biopsy**. The last thing you want is to find out your pet has a clotting problem after a chunk of the liver has been removed!

A small amount of ALT is present in red blood cells, and significant ALT elevations can occur if an animal is in a hemolytic crisis. As the red blood cells are being destroyed in an autoimmune state, the ALT is released into the bloodstream, just like bilirubin (as we discussed earlier in the Red Blood Cell story). These patients are obviously anemic as well. Profound, regenerative anemia plus ALT elevations should have you thinking of an immune crisis.

In certain breeds of dogs (Bedlington Terriers, West Highland White Terriers, and Dobermans) an increased ALT may indicate **copper storage disease**—where the body retains too much copper and deposits it into the liver. False elevations of ALT can result from **lipemia**, which is one reason fasting is recommended for routine lab work.

Conversely, the absence of ALT elevations does not mean that liver function is normal. Because the half-life on ALT is short, mild to moderate elevations may indicate that bloodwork was performed after the initial *insult* ("insult" is the medical term for an event which causes damage to a tissue or organ), and the numbers are on their way back down.

There is no clinical significance to decreased ALT values for the average *adult* animal. However, a rare condition called a **portosystemic** (or liver) **shunt** is sometimes seen in young animals when the normal blood supply to the liver does not develop properly and blood is re-routed around the liver. It is primarily a birth defect in young animals but can be an acquired problem in some cases. The "starved" liver will **atrophy** (wither and shrink), and the chemistry panel may exhibit a decreased ALT (along with a decreased BUN and **hypoglycemia**—low blood sugar). If the clinical signs of a liver shunt are present (stunted growth, failure to thrive, and unusual behavior after eating) along with abnormal lab values like these, your vet may recommend further diagnostic tests to rule out the possibility of a shunt.

ALKP or ALP (Alkaline Phosphatase)

This is an enzyme of induction—that is, rather than leaking out of affected liver cells during damage, this enzyme gets "turned on" by certain drugs and disease conditions. As a result, it is not as specific to the liver as ALT, since it can be influenced by a number of outside sources, but it is sensitive for certain types of liver problems.

- **ALKP (alkaline phosphatase): Normals vary with lab (the lab will provide ranges)**

Animals with healing bone fractures and rapidly growing large breed puppies can normally show ALKP elevations, and this isn't a cause for alarm. But significant elevations can be seen in diseases of the bone, such as bone cancer and infection of the bone (including severe dental disease). Significant elevations of ALKP can also be seen secondary to an inflammation of the pancreas and must be viewed in relation to what the pancreatic values are exhibiting.

ALKP is useful in detecting subtle cholestatic disease—**cholestasis** is the development of bile products in abnormal concentrations in the bloodstream. It can lead to **jaundice (icterus is the animal term)**, but as it is not the sole cause of icterus, cholestasis should not be used interchangeably with icterus. Animals with icterus typically have yellow mucous membranes: their gums and the whites of their eyes are bright yellow in color, like that of a banana. Anything that interferes with bile flow through the liver and into the intestines can cause cholestasis—such as gallstones, cancer of the liver, toxins or diseases that cause the liver to swell and close off bile ducts. ALKP values will start to increase long before there are clinical signs (such as weight loss, vomiting, liver enlargement, and an accumulation of fluid in the abdomen known as **ascites**).

In dogs, the major causes of significant elevations ALKP are liver disease, drug therapy (the use of steroids, phenobarbital, and barbiturates), diabetes mellitus, and **hyperadrenocorticism** (Cushing's disease). The magnitude of elevation does not correlate with the severity of disease, although elevations of greater than six times normal are suggestive of Cushing's disease in the dog. This syndrome must be ruled out through further, specialized testing.

Many older dogs have mild to moderately elevated levels of ALKP, which are age-related. Unless the ALKP levels are significantly elevated, I usually examine what medications they may be taking, look at diet, and monitor the blood levels for 1-2 months before becoming more aggressive in my diagnostics.

Bilirubin (Total Bilirubin: TBILI)

Bilirubin originates inside red blood cells and in the macrophages of the liver, spleen, and bone (that is, the large cells that remove "pathogens" such as tissue debris, bacteria, fungi, cancer cells...etc.). It binds to plasma proteins and is transported to the liver. There, it is converted to another form and secreted into the bile ducts.

- **Bilirubin: normal < 1.0 mg/dl**

In species that have them, the gallbladder acts as a reservoir for bile ("gall") storage until it can be secreted into the intestines during digestion. This bitter substance is the source behind the colorful expression of describing a person or situation as "galling."

A dog's gallbladder, by the way, does not empty unless the dog has consumed a meal. This is why some dogs who are fed only once daily, or who have skipped a meal, might vomit up bile and otherwise appear healthy and happy.

The bile pigments are responsible for the yellow color of vomit and the brown color of feces. Small amounts of bile are re-circulated and then deposited in the form of urobilinogen in the urine (also yellow). When there is **too much bilirubin** in the body, the excess spills first into the urine, which will turn bright orange/yellow, and then eventually the excess backs up into the bloodstream. At levels of 3-4 mg/dl, the mucous membranes and the whites of the eyes will appear visibly yellow. This condition is known as **icterus (jaundice** is the older term).

The two main causes of icterus are hemolytic disease (lysis of the red blood cells releases the plasma-bound bilirubin) and primary liver disease. The presence of bilirubin plus a regenerative anemia (and increased ALT) is suggestive of an autoimmune bleeding disorder. Any condition that disrupts bile flow will also result in an increased bilirubin. This can be due to many causes, such as bile duct obstruction due to tumor or gallstones, conditions of liver congestion (such as fatty liver disease or cholestatic disease), or conditions of liver scarring, such as cirrhosis. Dogs can often have severe liver disease before icterus is present.

Cats are particularly prone to a condition called fatty liver syndrome, in part because we here in the US tend to feed dry cat food instead of wet food. Cats are obligate carnivores, which means they must eat a protein-based diet, unlike dogs which can manage on a diet higher in carbs. Fatty liver syndrome is usually triggered when an overweight cat stops eating abruptly for whatever reason and begins to lose weight too rapidly, causing fat to be released into the blood, which is then mopped up by the liver. The liver becomes choked with the fat and ceases to function properly. Fatty liver disease is potentially reversible, but it requires the force-feeding of a high protein diet to reverse the trend. Many times, this requires the placement of a feeding tube and a liquid diet until the cat improves, which can be as long as a month or more.

Liver Values: Conclusion

You can see that despite the cause, the liver enzymes tend to react in a similar fashion to a wide variety of insults (damage-causing events). Sometimes, a liver biopsy is necessary to determine the underlying problem and affect necessary treatment.

Often, because a patient is not a suitable candidate for surgical biopsy at the time of presentation, abnormalities of the liver are treated first symptomatically with fluids and antibiotics until the patient is more stable. If after such treatment, the liver values are not improving, further diagnostics are warranted. As I mentioned before, because the liver is also responsible for secreting many of the blood clotting factors, **it is always advisable to run a clotting profile BEFORE surgical biopsy on an animal with suspected liver disease**. (Remember what I said about repeating important things?)

Section 3.3: The Pancreatic Values

The pancreas serves the body in two ways:

- as an **endocrine** organ, it secretes hormones directly into the blood; and

- as an **exocrine** organ it secretes enzymes through a duct, rather directly into the blood.

Most people are familiar with the endocrine role of the pancreas in the production of insulin and the regulation of blood sugar. In a moment, we're going to look in detail at diabetes—the condition when this system fails.

In its exocrine role, the pancreas is also responsible for secreting certain digestive enzymes into the duodenum (upper small intestine). **Pancreatic insufficiency** is a condition where considerable damage or under-development of the organ has resulted in an inability to secrete these digestive enzymes in normal amounts and this causes a maldigestion syndrome, where your pet cannot digest food normally. This can occur because of **pancreatitis** (and inflammation of the pancreas) or may be hereditary in some dogs. German Shepherds are prone to maldigestion syndromes and pancreatic insufficiency.

Pancreatitis is an inflammation of the pancreas, which can be triggered by eating rich, fatty foods or by ingesting certain medications. In this situation, the pancreas, over-stimulated for whatever reason, begins pumping out digestive enzymes to such an extent that the pancreas itself is affected and becomes so inflamed that the enzymes may even begin to digest the pancreas itself. Symptoms can be anything from mild vomiting and diarrhea to an inability to keep any food or water down, along with intense abdominal pain.

Diabetes Mellitus (DM)

DM is a condition where either the pancreas produces an insufficient quantity of insulin to regulate blood sugar, or the body's insulin receptors are unable to respond appropriately (**insulin resistance**) to the insulin that is present. In the case of insulin resistance, because the receptors are no longer functioning properly, the body can't regulate blood glucose normally. This causes the liver to convert more glycogen to glucose to get more of it into the cells where it is needed as fuel. In both cases, the patients develop persistently elevated blood glucose levels, known as **hyperglycemia**.

Blood glucose elevations will result in the body dumping the excess glucose into the urine when the kidney threshold for blood glucose is reached, since the kidneys regulate the amount that should circulate through normally and send the rest to the urine. Diabetes is the most common cause of **glucosuria** (glucose in the urine), but there are other causes, such as stress, a recent large dose of steroids, or concurrent Cushing's disease. Glucosuria is **ALWAYS** grounds for checking a blood glucose level.

The normal glucose range for dogs is 80-120 mg/dl.

In Type 1 diabetes, the pancreas isn't making insulin. Providing insulin usually corrects the problem, as long as the proper diet is also maintained. Dogs tend to get Type 1 diabetes and are usually easy to regulate once the problem has been identified. Easy doesn't mean it doesn't require a lot of monitoring or special diets, it just means that dogs tend to respond in predictable manner to insulin supplementation. In dogs, diabetes is frequently secondary to a bout of severe pancreatitis, or from multiple small episodes of pancreatitis, which have damaged that organ. The pancreas becomes dysfunctional and doesn't produce enough insulin. Giving insulin injections usually corrects the problem.

Most of the dogs I see with diabetes have been fed from the table and are significantly overweight. I'm not talking about feeding a balanced, fresh cooked or raw diet, here. I'm referring to sliding the last bit of greasy, fried, fatty, or carb-rich food off your plate to your dog. Food we should be eating less of ourselves!

There are, however, certain breeds more prone to diabetes than others. Small dogs, and terriers in general, seem to be the most common patients I see with both pancreatitis and diabetes. Is it because they are more likely to be indulged with table food? Possibly. But mini-Schnauzers have an above average incidence of diabetes. This could have something to do with the fact that Schnauzers frequently have markedly elevated triglyceride levels and are the only dogs that sometimes need drugs to control cholesterol levels.

Cats, however, tend to get insulin-resistant diabetes, more like type 2 diabetes in humans. This can make them challenging to regulate, particularly if you aren't successful in getting them to eat special diets. Eating dry kibble, which tends to be too high in carbs for cats, leads to obesity and insulin resistance.

Due to the different types of diabetes in animals, certain kinds of injectable insulin may work better for one species than another. This is why your pet may not be able to use the same brand of insulin as someone else in your family.

Regulating Diabetes

When diabetes is present, your vet may perform a **blood glucose curve.** This is a series of blood sugar checks over a 12–24 hour period to get a picture of what the glucose is doing over time and in response to insulin therapy.

A more useful test to monitor the well-controlled diabetic may be the **serum fructosamine** levels. Serum fructosamine is related to blood glucose concentrations and reflects what the blood glucose levels have been doing over the past several weeks. It can help differentiate between real hyperglycemia and that which is stress-induced (by the vet visit, perhaps?). Serum fructosamine levels less than 400 mg/dl are associated with good control of the diabetes. I frequently use fructosamine levels to monitor diabetes in cats, as it tends to be less stressful on them than a blood glucose curve, but more on diabetes in cats in a moment.

Your vet may have you monitor at home the presence or absence of glucosuria in your pet using urine strips to help keep tract of the diabetes treatment but never use glucosuria to determine whether to change insulin administration! Urine glucose levels do not accurately reflect what is currently going on in the bloodstream (i.e., there is a "lag" time between what you have in the blood verses what you see in the urine). Monitoring the urine glucose levels should be used primarily to see how well-controlled the diabetes is between regular vet visits.

There are many diabetic pet management groups out there which may advocate purchasing a home glucometer and testing your pet's blood sugar yourself. Keep in mind that drugstore glucometers are designed to be used on humans and may not give you an accurate reading on your pet.

Regulation of a diabetic can depend on many factors. Some animals regulate easily while others do not. The development of infections, or the presence of another disease problem can greatly complicate the regulation process.

Uncontrolled Diabetes

Uncontrolled diabetes usually results in excessive weight loss, dehydration due to the body pulling water into the urine to dilute the sugar, and a high degree of susceptibility to infection. The energy drain that results in the dramatic weight loss associated with uncontrolled diabetes causes the formation of **ketones** in the blood and urine. (Ketones are also seen in any state resulting in starvation—like being shipwrecked on an island with nothing to eat!) **When the levels of ketones rise, the animal may develop ketoacidosis, a life-threatening condition that requires hospitalization, fluid therapy, and emergency reduction of the blood glucose levels to correct**. Ketoacidosis is a common condition in the uncontrolled diabetic dog.

Some animals with diabetes may suddenly develop cataracts, so if this happens to your pet, bloodwork to rule out diabetes is a good idea. About 30% of dogs with DM will develop cataracts within the first 5-6 months.

Diabetes in Cats

One of the things we frequently hear in veterinary medicine is that "cats are not small dogs." This is especially true when it comes to diabetes management. For one thing, cats are **obligate carnivores**. That means that they NEED to eat a high-protein, low carbohydrate diet. Cats originated in desert countries, and survived on a high-water content, high-protein content, small volume meal: mice. Dogs are more omnivorous as a carnivore, which means they tolerate a higher carbohydrate level in their food.

As I said above, dogs tend to get Type 1 diabetes. Cats, though, tend to get Type 2, insulin-resistant diabetes. Why? Because at the time of writing this text, nearly **all** dry cat food is TOO HIGH in carbs for cats! Cats need to eat a diet of 10% carbs or less, and most commercial cat food is around 15% carbs. There are a few companies that have created prescription "metabolic" dry diets for cats, so if your cat refuses to eat any wet food, you might want to consult with your veterinarian about healthier dry options. In addition, there are prescription diets aimed at helping to stabilize blood sugar levels in both dogs and cats. They are certainly worth investigating.

What happens when you consistently eat a diet too high in carbs for your body? Let's say you have that wonderful sugar-glazed doughnut for breakfast, and you wash it down with a soda. Because the high-fructose corn syrup in the soda is in a liquid form, your body can absorb it into the blood stream very quickly. That, combined with the doughnut, is going to shoot your blood sugar through the roof. Your pancreas, wanting to maintain your sugar within certain parameters, pumps out insulin to bring your blood sugar down.

But insulin is so effective at bringing the blood glucose down that now your blood sugar plummets. Your brain needs glucose to run effectively, so when your blood sugar gets low, you get irritable and have a tough time thinking clearly. If it gets too low, you might pass out or even have a seizure. So, the body has a strong self-protective mechanism to trigger hunger when this happens. You're at work, and it's several hours before you can eat lunch, so what do you do? You grab another sugary snack, and the roller coaster ride begins all over again. Chronic dieting can blunt this response, but for most of us, eating a high carb meal in the morning sets us up for an entire day of bouncing between high blood sugar and low blood sugar and eating to stay functional.

When you keep doing this, the insulin receptors in your pancreas eventually become deadened to the presence of insulin in your bloodstream. It begins to take more and more insulin to control your blood sugar, and eventually, the receptors become unresponsive to the amount of insulin your body can produce. That is how you develop Type 2 diabetes, and as an analogy, it also explains why cats fed dry food do so as well.

Feeding dry cat food is associated with a whole host of serious health problems along with diabetes: obesity, fatty liver syndrome, pancreatitis, an increased risk of cancer and heart disease, and joint problems. Cats that are obese develop a greasy stripe down the middle of their backs, along with dandruff and an inability to clean themselves properly, which can lead to urine scalding.

It can be prevented by **not** feeding your cat dry food.

We jokingly refer to this as the **Catkins Diet**, but I passionately believe for every dollar you spend on wet cat food, you will save it in medical bills. An all-canned (wet food) diet also keeps the urine pH where it is supposed to be, thus helping to prevent the development of crystals in the urine, which can lead to life-threatening urinary blockages in male cats. These problems can resolve when we change from a dry to an all-canned diet. Don't believe me? Google the "Catkins Diet."

I don't pretend it is always easy to change your cat's diet. In certain countries, feeding dry cat food is the norm. We tend to raise our cats on dry food, and it is certainly less expensive and easier to feed. Cats also have significantly fewer taste buds then other species, so they come by their "finicky" reputation honestly. I've never seen a dumpster cat be a picky eater, however. This is because they learned early in life to eat a wide variety of foods. Ironically, it is the cat who was well-cared for from kittenhood that often becomes locked in to eating only one or two foods.

Unlike other species, cats are not adaptable when it comes to food changes and will sometimes starve themselves than eat something they do not consider food. The last thing you want is for an overweight cat to go on a hunger strike — the section below on fatty liver syndrome explains why!

My advice? Offer both dry kibble and canned wet food to your growing kitten so it learns to eat both. Research your diets. Talk to your vet about the best food choices. I am not an advocate of home cooking or raw diets for your cat because cats have extremely specific amino acid requirements from their food, and if they do not get it in their diets, they will steal it from their heart tissue and other important places. I once had a vegetarian client who insisted on feeding her cat a vegetarian diet. Her cat had significant—and entirely preventable—cardiomyopathy as a result. The client refused to listen to any nutritional advice. Given her stance, an herbivore would have made a better pet for her.

Keep in mind two things when talking with your veterinarian, however:

- First, most veterinarians get their information on nutrition from the big pet food companies. This is partly because these companies usually make prescription diets that are important to managing serious disease conditions. While I believe in the value of specially designed diets to treat a whole host of medical problems, I recognize that my education in this matter has been biased. I try to make sure I stay up to date on the latest information from a wide variety of legitimate sources.

- Second, just because a company has cute commercials touting the wonders and benefits of their foods, this doesn't mean their product is a good one. Likewise, just because a recommended diet is promoted as being "natural" doesn't make it necessarily healthy for your pet. It should be understood that what someone says on social media isn't necessarily a legitimate source too.

The most crucial factors in obesity in cats include:

- Most people in the U.S. feed dry food exclusively.

- Most people allow their cats access to food 24/7.

- For safety reasons, many cats are 100% indoors.

So, what should you do? Not all cats can or will make the switch to an all-canned diet. The taste window closes early in a cat's life, and they are reluctant to try new foods after a certain age. I think, for some cats, they won't touch canned food because they don't believe it *is* food. Because of this, they will make themselves seriously ill if you do a "you will eat this or else" approach to feeding them. Hunger strikes, especially in obese cats, can trigger life-threatening fatty liver syndrome, as we've mentioned before.

So, I recommend all cats be offered a combination of canned plus dry food as kittens. To be perfectly honest, I believe that young cats should be started out on canned food only, but I do recognize there are times when feeding some dry is necessary. If a cat isn't used to eating dry kibble, however, a sudden influx (while you're on vacation, or you get snowed in and have few options) might result in an upset stomach, so it's not a bad idea to give your cat a little dry food on a regular basis. When I say "some dry" however, I mean a pinch of dry kibble, and only if the cat is not diabetic or struggling with weight issues. This should be an excellent quality dry food, and you should not leave heaping bowls of food around the house for the cat to access 24 hours a day.

Some cats truly prefer dry food, and it is difficult, if not impossible, to get them to eat wet/canned food. I recommend you continue to offer it, as you may hit upon a flavor or consistency they like. It is also critical that if you must feed dry kibble that you do NOT simply fill a bowl or a gravity-type feeder and walk away. Not only can free choice feeding like this lead to a whole host of medical issues, but I also see behavioral problems arise from this habit as well. My current house cat doesn't tolerate any dry food. It makes him vomit. I have some feral cats (trapped, neutered, vaccinated, and released) that I feed twice daily: ¼ cup of dry kibble each. Not only are they maintaining a decent weight, and I'm decreasing the risk of them developing a medical problem that would be difficult to treat, but I'm not feeding the entire raccoon and possum population in the neighborhood as well.

If I am trying to regulate a new diabetic cat, or if I need to get some weight off a cat safely, I recommend a gradual change to an all-canned diet. In general, any flavor is okay, but I try to avoid fish. Many cats are allergic to fish (and when you think about it, how often would the average cat have access to fish if we didn't give it to them?). Moreover, there may be a correlation between eating canned fish and the development of hyperthyroidism in older cats, so I try to avoid feeding anything that lists fish in the top five ingredients. Polybrominated diphenyl ethers (PBDEs), which researchers have found to be elevated in blood samples of hyperthyroid cats, are also higher in canned fish. Fish is a common filler in cat food, so it might be tough to find something completely fish-free.

The average ten-pound cat should eat one half of a tuna-fish sized can of food (5.5 ounces) twice daily, according to Deborah Greco, DVM, Ph.D., a leading researcher in the field of feline diabetes and, at one time, an internist and endocrinologist at The Animal Medical Center in New York. This is the equivalent of two Fancy Feast sized cans (or two 3.3-ounce pouches). A fifteen-pound cat would eat 1.5 of the tuna-fish sized cans, a twenty-pound cat would eat two tuna-fished sized cans. That sounds like a lot, particularly if you're putting your cat on a diet, but the important thing with overweight cats is that we do not trigger fatty liver syndrome! This also presumes that the cat isn't eating any dry food at all by this point.

Fatty liver syndrome is when the body enters a state of starvation, and the body begins to release fat stores to make them available for fuel. Unfortunately, if you have an overweight animal, there is a lot of fat available, and it floods the bloodstream, where the liver blots it up like a sponge. The fat chokes out the liver and causes organ failure. It can be reversed but only with aggressive treatment, so it is best to avoid it altogether. A tubby tabby who doesn't eat for more than 24 hours is at risk of fatty liver syndrome, so if your cat isn't eating, you need to get him checked out by your vet, ASAP!

If your cat has never eaten canned food before, make the introductions S-L-O-W-L-Y. Offer the canned food in a separate dish from the dry. If your cat refuses to eat the canned food, it might avoid any dry that touched it as well. Start with a small spoonful of the canned food. If your cat eats it, then each day offer a little more canned and a little less dry, making the transition over a period of about two to three weeks.

Many people complain they can't feed a set portion of food twice a day in a multi-cat household, as one cat will get more than its fair share. I feed all my cats in carriers. They expect to be fed there; they run into the carriers as I get the bowls ready. I shut them in with their food and they clean it up on the spot. Ten minutes tops, and the cats are ready to be let out again. It makes life so much simpler—not to mention, I have no trouble getting my cats into carriers when they need to leave the house!

If you have a diabetic cat, any changes in diet must be made slowly and under a veterinarian's supervision! I'm going to repeat this: **If you have a diabetic cat any changes in diet must be made slowly and under a veterinarian's supervision!** You can run into serious problems with crashing blood sugar as your cat's insulin needs change during diet modification, and your vet needs to be on board with these changes.

Hypoglycemia: when blood glucose levels are too low

Even though the body does not tolerate persistently elevated glucose levels without profound consequences, it is even less tolerant of blood glucose levels that are BELOW normal. We've all experienced that feeling of light-headedness when we haven't eaten in a while. (It would be better to say that some of us have; others of us have become surly and grumpy when dinner has been delayed too long...)

This is the body's way of warning you that you need to re-fuel soon OR ELSE. Ever wondered what the "or else" would look like? The brain has an extremely high demand for readily available glucose. Conditions that result in hypoglycemia can cause fainting or even seizures. If you ever have a diabetic pet that is being treated with insulin, and you find your pet in a stuporous or collapsing state, rub honey or Karo syrup on the gums and contact your vet (or an after-hours clinic) on an emergency basis. **Hypoglycemia, if uncorrected, can be fatal**. If you are ever uncertain as to whether to administer your pet's usual insulin dose, and your vet is not available for consult, it is better to skip a dose than not. But consult your vet whenever possible!

Hypoglycemia can also be seen in other situations as well. Sometimes hunting dogs can burn up all their available blood glucose in cold field trial situations, and many sport dog trainers carry high-calorie supplements with them during sporting events. Toy breed dogs, especially as puppies, can sometimes develop hypoglycemia if they aren't getting fed frequently. There is also an insulin-producing tumor that will cause the patient's blood sugar to repeatedly bottom out. Puppies with parvo can also develop hypoglycemia due to the intestinal and inability to keep food down. Hypoglycemia can also occur when there is severe infection in the body, and the body keeps utilizing the available glucose to feed the cells fighting off the infection.

NEWSFLASH

> Remember: low blood sugar will kill you faster than high blood sugar will.

Amylase (AMYL) and Lipase (LIP)

Amylase is one of the digestive enzymes secreted by the salivary glands in the mouth and by the exocrine function of the pancreas. Because the salivary glands begin secreting amylase in anticipation of digesting food, sometimes if you have a pet recovering from pancreatitis, your vet may recommend that you isolate them from areas of the house where food prep is taking place, as the smell of cooking may trigger release of additional amylase.

Amylase (AMYL): Normals vary with lab

Elevations of amylase are seen with kidney and pancreatic disease. Mild to moderate elevations (less than two times normal range) are usually seen in kidney dysfunctions that result in decreased filtration, so the "elevation" of amylase is due to the decreased filtration rate and not because the production of amylase has increased. Marked elevations are usually indicative of pancreatic disease (such as an inflammation of the pancreas), but the level of elevation does not always correlate well with the severity of disease. Amylase levels also do not necessarily rise when pancreatic disease is present. There is little clinical significance to low amylase values.

Lipase (LIP) is a pancreatic enzyme that catalyzes the breakdown of fats to fatty acids and glycerol or other alcohols.

Lipase (LIP): Normals vary with lab

Lipase levels rise under the same conditions that cause amylase levels to increase. Lipase levels may be more specific for pancreatic disease than amylase, however. Again, like amylase, the levels do not necessarily rise whenever pancreatic disease is present, nor do levels correlate with the severity of disease.

Elevated lipase levels in a dog showing abdominal pain and vomiting, however, should be taken seriously. Pancreatitis has the potential to be life-threatening if not treated appropriately. There is now a tableside snap test available to test for canine lipase levels, which can be very useful in determining if pancreatitis is present. A positive test correlates with pancreatitis.

There is no clinical significance to low values.

The presence of amylase and lipase elevations **together** is usually an indication of pancreatic disease but often must be viewed in consideration with both the liver and kidney values to help rule in/rule out the pancreas as the source of the problem. As the absence of elevated values does not necessarily rule out a pancreatic problem, further diagnostics (such as abdominal ultrasound) may be indicated when pancreatic abnormalities are suspected. In a case of pancreatitis, the ALKP and white cell counts may be elevated as well as the pancreatic enzymes.

Chronic pancreatitis might not reveal any abnormalities on lab work because the pancreas is too severely damaged to secrete enzymes anymore. Chronic pancreatitis frequently leads to diabetes and is often the result of eating high-carb, high-fat diets that burn the pancreas up over time. Animals in the wild don't typically eat high fat, high carb diets, although exceptions are made. During the cycles of the 17-year cicadas, in the years that the cicadas emerge, many animals gorge on the calorie-dense insects. Wildlife experts report bumper crops of baby animals in these years, as the parents have plenty of food to eat. In fact, some dogs find cicadas so delicious, we've seen them pack on the pounds in those seasons, so try not to let your pet eat too many!

NEWSFLASH

Elevations of pancreatic enzymes can occur in other conditions besides primary pancreatic disease

Case Study: Michelob

Please bear in mind that bloodwork (or medical cases) rarely falls into neat little categories. There can be multiple problems going on at one time, but for the sake of simplifying our discussion, I am going to present an uncomplicated case example.

Michelob is a six-year-old lab cross. He is markedly overweight at one hundred pounds, but records indicate a dramatic weight loss of sixteen pounds within the last three months. He is drinking lots of water and urinating frequently. He is not vomiting, but he is not eating well, either. On presentation he is notably dehydrated, and he has cataracts in both eyes.

Mic's bloodwork shows his CBC is within normal limits. His Chem Profile looks like this:

Test	Results	Reference Range	Units
Albumin (ALB)	3.01	2.7-4.4	g/dl
Alkaline phosphatase (ALKP)	100	5-131	U/L
Alanine transferase (ALT)	60	12-118	U/L

Test	Results	Reference Range	Units
Amylase (AMYL)	753	500-1500	U/L
Blood Urea Nitrogen (BUN)	40 (H)	6-25	mg/dl
Calcium (Ca)	10.92	8.9-11.4	mg/dl
Cholesterol (CHOL)	400.2 (H)	92-324	mg/dl
Creatinine (CREA)	1.19	0.5-1.8	mg/dl
Glucose (GLU)	486.3 (H)	70-138	mg/dl
Phosphorus (PHOS)	4.75	2.5-6.0	mg/dl
Total bilirubin (TBILI)	0.8	0.00-0.90	mg/dl
Total Protein (TP)	8.9 (H)	5.2-8.2	g/dl
Globulins (GLOB)	4.99	2.5-4.5	g/dl

There would seem to be several things going on here, but we can show how they are all related:

- The most significant finding is that Mic is **hyperglycemic**. Such a high glucose reading is probably real and not due to stress or a recent injection of steroids, but the presence of glucose in the urine as well will help confirm the diagnosis of diabetes.

- The mild elevation of BUN could be related to dehydration (especially since the creatinine levels are normal). Checking the urine specific gravity and finding it very concentrated (greater than 1.050) would confirm this.

- A urinalysis is necessary to determine if ketones are present in the urine as well, as this would indicate a more serious condition: **ketoacidosis**, which might require hospitalization and aggressive treatment to correct. Finding sugar in the urine would also show that the elevated blood sugar is a real finding and has been going on for a while now.

- The elevated cholesterol levels could be related to the diabetes, but Mic might also be **hypothyroid** (another common cause of elevated cholesterol levels). Hypothyroidism could also explain (part) of his obesity problem. A thyroid test is indicated at this time.

- The increased total protein and globulins are also probably due to dehydration.

With aggressive therapy and regulation of his diabetes, Mic's condition may be managed for the rest of his life.

Section 3.4: The Electrolytes

Many of us were taught in high school biology class that a solution of salt water will conduct electricity. What you may not know is that electrolytes are salts contained within our bodily fluids and that they that move throughout the tissues. The cells have little pumps that manage the orderly movement of sodium (Na+) and potassium (K+) across the cell membranes to create the energy needed to run the cells (and all life). These **cations** (positively charged ions, like sodium) and **anions** (negatively charged ions, such as chloride) combine with minerals to create salts so that the minerals can move between reserve pools (for example in the bones) and circulate freely in the blood by "catching a ride" with the electrolytes.

The cells are so dependent on properly working Na/K pumps that the range for normal electrolyte levels is VERY narrow. Anything that disturbs fluid balance (vomiting, diarrhea, kidney dysfunction...etc.) will alter electrolyte levels. Because the body has such a narrow tolerance for alterations in electrolyte imbalances, dangerous excesses or deficiencies can result in life-threatening conditions. Weakness and collapse can be seen with electrolyte disturbances.

Potassium (K+)

Potassium: normal (3.8-5.8 mEq/L)

Potassium is an essential mineral and electrolyte involved in muscle contractions, heart function, and regulating water balance. It is obtained through eating.

Low Potassium Levels

Animals that are **anorexic,** (not eating) for whatever reason, may have low potassium levels. Certain medications, such as some common diuretics, may cause excess potassium loss into the urine. Kidney dysfunction can also result in potassium wasting.

The most common causes of low potassium are anorexia (failure to eat) and fluid loss. Anything that results in excess fluid being depleted from the body (in the form of excessive urination, vomiting, diarrhea, or burns covering large areas of skin) can result in potassium loss. The use of diuretics, especially those which do not spare potassium levels, may deplete the body's sources. Insulin administration, large IV doses of penicillin, steroids, aspirin, and administration of IV glucose can all result in a *shift* of potassium from the circulating blood to the interior of the tissue cells (**translocation**). Translocation can result in seriously low potassium levels initially, but caution must be used in correcting it, because the potassium is still *there,* just not readily available now.

A special mention should be made of diabetic dogs in a ketoacidotic crisis: they can present initially with normal or elevated potassium levels while they are in the ketoacidotic state, but the potassium levels can drop dramatically once the blood sugar levels are corrected and the cells take up more potassium from the blood stream (also a form of **translocation**). Such a patient may need frequent monitoring of electrolytes while on IV fluids to ensure that they receive appropriate fluid types or supplementation.

As far as cats are concerned, one of the most common problems we see in elderly cats with kidney issues is **hypokalemia**. Without the necessary potassium levels, the muscles can be so weak that these cats can't walk properly or hold up their heads. Supplementing with potassium, either in the diet or through fluids, is necessary to keep these cats mobile and healthy.

If you have ongoing fluid losses (such as serum weeping from severely burned skin or kidney failure resulting in excessive urinations, then giving potassium-deficient fluids (i.e., Lactated Ringers) as a replacement will also deplete potassium levels. Potassium levels are also typically decreased in early to moderate stages of kidney failure.

Sometimes you can get false decreases in potassium levels. This can be due to such conditions as lipemia (free fat in the blood), elevated BUN levels, toxic levels of theophylline (chocolate poisoning), and blood glucose levels greater than 1000mg/dl (severe hyperglycemia, usually because of uncontrolled diabetes).

High Potassium Levels

The most common causes of high potassium levels are increased intake (massive salt ingestion or IV administration of salt solutions), decreased output (end-stage renal failure or urinary blockage), and Addison's disease (**hyperadrenocorticism**).

Hypoadrenocorticism is a rare disease in which the body does not produce the trace amounts of steroids and glucocorticoids necessary to run the body and keep the electrolytes in balance. In addition to having markedly elevated potassium levels, these dogs also have exceptionally low sodium levels. Addisonian dogs often present on emergency with profound vomiting and diarrhea. Because they are experiencing fluid loss, they are frequently given IV fluids. They miraculously recover and look great because the electrolytes have been corrected. However, they soon will be out of balance again because the body is failing to maintain the correct levels. We often look at the sodium–potassium (Knack) ratio when trying to determine if a dog is Addisonian or not. Typically, dogs with Addison's have a Knack ratio of less than 27:1 unless fluids or steroids have been given.

Addison's disease is a rare finding in the general dog population—although standard poodles may have a hereditary predisposition—but it should be suspected any time you have electrolyte abnormalities. Some dogs with Addison's can present with back pain and signs of kidney compromise, which might lead to a misdiagnosis of disc disease or kidney failure. Be sure to look at the electrolytes too!

Markedly elevated potassium levels can also occur when the urinary tract is blocked, and urine is unable to leave the body (because of a bladder stone lodged in the urethra of a male dog or a male cat with urinary crystals, for example). The kidney values will also become severely elevated as well, but that's because there is a blockage in the filter, causing waste products to accumulate to toxic levels. If you can relieve the blockage in time, most animals will return to normal kidney function, and the electrolytes will stabilize.

There are conditions that can cause false increases as well: extremely high platelet counts (>100,000/mm3) or WBC counts >200,000/mm3 in blood samples that have been allowed to clot may release intracellular potassium into the blood sample. Abnormal cells, like leukemia cells, can also do the same. **Akitas have enough intracellular potassium that hemolysis during sampling** (fracturing of the RBC during the withdrawing of blood from the vein to the collection tube) **can result in falsely elevated levels in this breed**.

As lab testing equipment becomes more sophisticated, errors in handling the blood sample, such as creating hemolysis during sampling, will show up more frequently and is not necessarily breed-specific.

NEWSFLASH

If potassium levels are high enough, they WILL kill your pet. Back in the old days, before the creation of more humane euthanasia solutions, the common method of euthanizing an animal was to administer a potassium chloride solution IV. Elevated potassium levels interfere with your heart's ability to beat properly and stop the heart. Elevated potassium levels, either because of Addison's disease or an inability to urinate, is a critical situation that must be dealt with on an emergency basis!

Sodium (Na+)

Sodium: normal (141-154 mEq/L)

Sodium (Na+) is the main component of the Na+/K+ pump that works inside every cell to create and transport the energy needed to survive. It is essential for normal muscle and nerve functions and helps keep body fluids in balance.

Conditions that can alter the sodium values include the following: primarily drugs that alter fluid balance, non-steroidal anti-inflammatories (NSAIDs) and other chemotherapy drugs.

Low Sodium Levels

Causes of low sodium levels are excessive fluid loss through urination, vomiting, or diarrhea. Over-hydration, or the administration of electrolyte deficient IV fluids (ex. 5% dextrose in water, or Lactated Ringers), can also result in lowered sodium levels. This is not to say there is never an indication for using these types of fluids! Just that electrolytes may need to be monitored during the administration of such fluids.

Anything that decreases effective circulating blood volume, such as right-sided heart failure or liver cirrhosis, will also affect sodium levels by triggering the release of **antidiuretic hormone (ADH)**. If the body thinks the blood volume is low, either because it is truly low or because the heart isn't pumping strongly, then ADH will kick in so that you'll urinate less, and thus keep the blood pressure up. Because ADH causes water retention, the sodium concentration is effectively diluted out in the blood. Other conditions that affect ADH levels, such as hypothyroidism, will do the same.

Sodium levels can be depleted to due excessive vomiting, or because the bladder is ruptured (and the sodium is being lost into the abdomen, along with everything else in the urine), diarrhea (for some reason in particular, diarrhea associated with whipworm infection, probably because the whips live in the colon, and that's where a lot of water absorption takes place). Mild **hyponatremia** (low sodium levels) is common, and not necessarily of concern.

High Sodium Levels

Causes of high sodium levels include the following: excessive dehydration, excessive administration of salt without access to water (including hand-raised puppies with improperly mixed formulas), and sometimes the medications used to treat Addison's disease. Diabetes mellitus can cause an **osmotic diuresis**—a condition where to dilute the sugary urine, the body dumps lots of water into the urinary system. This can result in severe dehydration, as can undiagnosed kidney failure.

Chloride (Cl-)

Chloride: normal (105-115mEq/L)

Chloride (Cl-) is responsible for maintaining the acid-base (pH) balance in the body, regulating fluids, and transmitting nerve impulses. It is a negatively charged ion (anion) that binds to positively charged ions (cations) to create a salt, so anything that causes sodium losses tends to cause chloride losses as well.

Low Cl- levels are caused by diuretics, laxatives, the same fluid losses as with sodium, or large IV doses of penicillin-class drugs. The two most common causes of major decreases are vomiting and hypoadrenocorticism (Addison's disease). A **false decrease** may be due to lipemia (free fat in the bloodstream) or hemolysis, as well as vigorous exercise.

High Cl- levels are caused by the same things that cause sodium to go up. (Don't forget that table salt is NaCl—they go together!). The most common cause is dehydration. **False increases** may result due to colored pigments in the blood (hemoglobin, bilirubin) that may alter test results that depend on a color change.

NEWSFLASH

Electrolytes have a very narrow range for normal values.

Abnormalities of potassium levels can be life-threatening.

Anything that causes fluid losses can disturb electrolyte balance.

Animals with kidney disease are at elevated risk for severe imbalances, especially if something interferes with their ability to consume water.

Section 3.5: Miscellaneous Tests in the Chem Profile

These miscellaneous tests are of real importance in certain, specific instances. They will be included on most serum chemistry profiles and should always be considered when evaluating lab work but tend to play more of a supporting role than act as the main stars already discussed. You might want to save this section for when the subject comes up (or if you are an insomniac searching for a solution to your sleeplessness!).

Albumin

Albumin: Normal (2.3-3.9 g/dl)

Albumin is the largest protein that circulates in the bloodstream. It has several essential functions, including the binding of certain salts and minerals to its surface for transport within the body. It is too large to get through the filtration system of a healthy kidney glomerulus, and therefore, its size and presence helps maintain **oncotic pressure** in the blood. This is the pressure that keeps your plasma inside your blood vessels. Without normal albumin levels, fluids leak out of the vessels and weep across the liver, resulting in **edema** (fluid within the tissues of the skin and lungs) as well as **ascites** (free fluid in the abdomen).

Albumin can be lost through the GI tract because of parasites, GI ulceration or bleeding, and protein-losing enteropathies. It can also be lost through the urinary system through glomerular damage—part of the kidney filtering system. Another potential source of albumin loss is through the skin if there are massive burn injuries where serous fluid weeps openly from the burned tissue. Albumin can also be low from inadequate protein intake and from liver disease because the body isn't making enough, but usually low albumin levels serious enough to cause clinical signs are the result of loss rather than decreased production. Low albumin levels indicate a need for further testing: a fecal analysis to rule out parasites, a urinalysis to look for protein losses...etc.

Calcium

Calcium: Normal (8.5-11 mg/dl)

(Dogs less than one year old or giant breed puppies can go higher.)

Calcium is a mineral essential for healthy bones and teeth. It also has a role to play in blood clotting, muscle contraction, normal heart rhythm regulation, and nerve functions.

Low Calcium Levels

Hypocalcemia (decreased calcium levels in the bloodstream) is a common laboratory finding in dogs. Low albumin levels (hypoalbuminemia) are thought to be the major cause for this finding and there is a correction factor that vets use that will often adjust calcium levels back into a normal range. While there are a lot of causes for true low calcium levels, the practical list of things that can cause problems is short. After hypoalbuminemia, there is kidney failure (acute, chronic, and secondary to antifreeze poisoning), primary and secondary hypoparathyroidism (see below), and eclampsia (see below). Hypoparathyroidism, pancreatitis, and malabsorption syndromes are uncommon causes of low calcium levels.

Clinical signs of hypocalcemia include **tetany** (uncontrolled muscle spasm), weakness, or seizures. **Severe hypocalcemia can be life-threatening**. Treatment is a SLOW IV infusion of calcium—rapid infusion can be fatal. In some cases, long term calcium and vitamin D supplements may be indicated.

Primary hypoparathyroidism (HPT) is usually due to the destruction of the parathyroid gland, either through abnormal tissue growth (neoplasia, also known as cancer) or infiltration of the gland with lymphatic tissue. Secondary HPT is usually due to removal of a parathyroid tumor and is self-limiting when there is enough gland left to regenerate. The parathyroid gland can also be damaged during removal of a thyroid tumor (these glands sit directly on top of the thyroid glands) resulting in the same (usually self-limiting) decreased calcium levels.

Eclampsia (dangerously low blood calcium levels in nursing bitches) is seen primarily in small breed bitches with large litters during the period of greatest milk production (2-4 weeks post whelping) but can occur in a wide variety of pregnant dogs and can be seen pre-delivery as well.

High Calcium Levels

A single high calcium value should be confirmed by a second sample, as unexplained increases can sometimes be seen. A sustained elevation needs to be worked up. There may be no clinical signs directly associated with elevated calcium levels, or there may be vomiting and diarrhea.

The condition of **hyperparathyroidism** is one in which the parathyroid gland—a tiny little gland that is located near the thyroid gland—begins secreting an unusual amount of calcitriol and parathyroid hormones that help regulate calcium balance in the body.

Hypercalcemia of malignancy is the number one cause of persistent, markedly elevated calcium levels. All the other causes of hypercalcemia are uncommon.

The most common cause for hypercalcemia in dogs is cancer, and the most common cancers associated with this syndrome are lymphosarcoma or adenocarcinomas (such as mammary or anal gland tumors, as well as other carcinomas, and multiple myeloma). After cancer has been ruled out, the other (infrequent) causes of elevated calcium are Addison's disease, kidney failure, primary hyperparathyroidism, an overdose of Vitamin D (either in rat poison, plants, or accidental ingestion of human supplements), and diseases of the bones resulting in **lysis** (such as fungal disease, bone infection...etc.). Lysis is the disintegration or destruction of tissues, such as cells or bone.

Some tumors are capable of secreting bone-resorption factors which cause the bone near a tumor (and more distantly as well) to undergo lysis. These factors (and others) may act on the bone directly or in the intestines and kidneys to alter calcium metabolism and result in increased circulating levels. This condition can result in **pseudo hyperparathyroidism** (to distinguish it from primary tumors of the parathyroid gland), but although the syndromes may seem similar on lab work, primary hyperparathyroidism is rare.

False increases may occur in lipemic or hemolyzed (that's when the red blood cells get fractured during the blood draw) samples—as we've seen for many other lab values already. The use of the anticoagulant EDTA can falsely increase or decrease calcium levels, depending on the method of analysis. It is important to rule these factors out because there are not many causes of hypercalcemia.

There is a condition in cats called **idiopathic hypercalcemia**, which means the pathology of the syndrome is not clearly understood. These cats typically drink excessive amounts of water and urinate excessively as well, but the unusual amount of calcium in their systems makes them very prone to life-threatening urinary blockages due to the formation of calcium stones in their urinary systems. Initially, other causes of hypercalcemia need to be ruled out before calling it idiopathic. Treatment is the most successful when it occurs prior to significant organ damage.

Phosphorus

Phosphorus: normal (2.5-5.5 mg/dl)

(Young dogs and giant breeds may exceed 2x normal)

Phosphorus in the body is essential for a tissue and cell growth, maintenance, and repair. It's also essential in the production of the genetic building blocks, DNA and RNA.

Like calcium (see above), values can be affected by lipemia and hemolysis.

Low phosphorus levels caused by the **combination** of **elevated calcium** and **decreased phosphorous** are only seen in cases of hypercalcemia of malignancy and hyperparathyroidism. Another cause of decreased phosphorous (alone) is ketoacidosis in diabetes mellitus.

High phosphorus levels are seen in azotemia/kidney failure, hyperthyroidism (primarily seen in cats; rarely seen in dogs), nutritional imbalances, an overdose of vitamin D, and hypoparathyroidism.

NEWSFLASH

> If calcium is HIGH and phosphorous LOW--rule out
> cancer
>
> If both calcium and phosphorous are elevated, check out
> kidney function.

Cholesterol

Cholesterol: normal (80-300mg/dl)

Cholesterol is waxy substance found in the bloodstream. Cholesterol is needed by the body to make hormones, vitamin D, and substances that help digestion.

There are four major causes of increased cholesterol:

- Hypothyroidism: a condition in which the thyroid gland doesn't produced enough hormones (underactive thyroid)

- Cushing's disease: a condition caused by an excess of the hormone cortisol (see Section 11 for more information). Many **Cushingoid** dogs have elevated cholesterol levels because they are also concurrently diabetic because of their primary hormonal disease. In the absence of lab work supporting diabetes or kidney failure, a thyroid test should be run on all dogs with elevated cholesterol levels.

- Diabetes mellitus: a condition we discussed in depth in section 3.3 on pancreatic values.

- Nephrotic syndrome, which is a term used to describe a series of laboratory findings: markedly elevated urine proteins (indicating loss of proteins into the urine), lipiduria (fat in the urine), hyperlipidemia (elevated fat levels in the blood—the blood will often appear "milky"), and peripheral edema (the limbs will swell as the body will be unable to keep fluid within the blood vessels, due to the loss of proteins). Nephrotic syndrome occurs when the normal architecture of the kidney has been replaced by an abnormal protein.

False increases can be caused by jaundice (icterus) or by steroids. Lipemia may result in inaccurate values.

Decreased cholesterol is rarely a problem, although it may be seen in maldigestion/malabsorption/malnutrition syndromes.

Triglycerides

Triglycerides: normal (10-150 mg/dl)

Triglycerides are a type of fat (lipid) found in the blood.

Increased levels are usually associated with grossly lipemic serum— usually in the blood of a non-fasted patient. If it persists on a fasted blood sample, rule out diabetes, starvation, and hypothyroidism. Increased levels can also be seen in acute pancreatitis and in Schnauzers with **idiopathic hyperlipidemia** (*idiopathic* means of unknown origin or cause. I remember this term by saying, "the idiots don't understand the pathology." (Make sure your vet has a sense of humor before using the word in this manner!) Pancreatitis can be a life-threatening situation, so you need to take hyperlipidemia seriously until proven otherwise.

Globulins

Globulins are proteins that circulate in the blood and perform numerous functions. Except for the immunoglobulins, most globulins are synthesized and stored in the liver. When electrophoresis is used to separate out the globulins for examination, certain patterns of increases are seen with certain types of disease. Hyperglobulinemia is seen in some types of liver/biliary disease.

A **gammopathy** refers to a disorder that results in proliferation of the immunoglobulins. There are two types of gammopathies:

- **monoclonal,** where there is an excess of one type of heavy or light chain immunoglobulins. Monoclonal gammopathies are associated with lymphocytic/plasmocytic disorders such as multiple myeloma (MM), lymphosarcoma, and occasionally infectious diseases such as Ehrlichia. It is important to remember that MM and Ehrlichia both can have monoclonal gammopathies and suppressed bone marrow function, so additional testing needs to be done if this is present.

- **polyclonal,** where two or more heavy chains and both types of light chains are involved. Polyclonal gammopathies include chronic inflammation (bacterial, fungal, and rickettsial disease), parasitism (including demodex and heartworms), cancer and some types of immune mediated disease (such as feline infectious peritonitis in cats).

Newborns have typically 60-80% of normal adult globulin values, which is one of the reasons passive transfer of maternal antibodies in colostrum (the mother's first milk) is so important to the survival of baby animals. Animals with combined immunodeficiency disorders rarely survive to weaning—succumbing to viral infections such as distemper or parvo. Low globulin levels can also result from liver insufficiency.

Section 4: Concluding Thoughts on the CBC and Chemistry Profile

That was a great deal of information to take in but remember that everything we've looked at in the earlier sections covers only the **basic** tests carried out in a CBC and chemistry profile (or "panel"). Your veterinarian may want to perform additional tests based on the findings of this basic lab work, such as a urinalysis, fecal analysis, heartworm testing, or more specific liver function tests, such as a bile acid analysis. We'll look at those in more detail in the following sections.

Hopefully, now you can see how the interpretation of one test result must be viewed in relation to other test results and any clinical signs your pet may or may not be showing. By now, I think you'll have realized there are limitations as well as benefits to doing basic lab work, since lab work doesn't necessarily tell you everything.

Normal lab work does not necessarily mean the animal is in optimal health. It is possible to have serious disease present in the body and have normal lab work. Diseases of the central nervous or musculoskeletal system, as well as certain types of cancer or primary gastrointestinal disease, may not be revealed in a minimum database analysis.

It is also important to realize just how hard the body will work to keep mineral values in the normal range, resorting to stealing resources from bones, if necessary, to do so. Just because your pet's lab work appears normal, this does not prove you are feeding a healthy and balanced diet! If you're not sure whether your home-cooked or raw diet is balanced— run an analysis on the diet, not the dog!

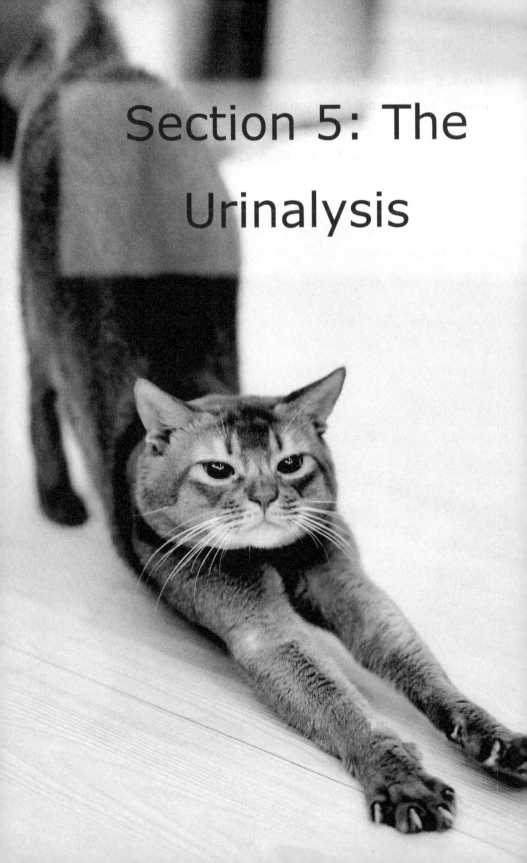

Section 5: The Urinalysis

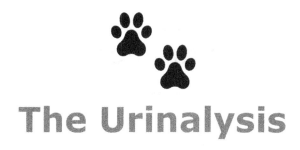

The Urinalysis

The urinalysis is an important but often overlooked part of the MDB. Examination of the urine can sometimes identify health issues before chemical changes register in the bloodstream or become clinically apparent in your dog. In cases of urinary tract infections, sometimes the only positive lab findings will be in the urine sample. Dietary imbalances can lead to elevated urinary pH and crystals in the urine before any other health issues show up.

Section 5.1: Collecting Samples

Urine samples can be collected in a variety of ways. Sometimes your vet will insist on collection via one method over another because the manner of collection can affect results.

One important note: no matter how the urine sample is collected, for the most accurate results, the sample should be examined within an hour of collection. After that time, bacteria and crystals may start to form that were not necessarily present in the fresh sample and skew the results.

Free Catch Method

There are many times when a "free catch" sample is entirely appropriate. This is a sample caught in a clean container while the dog is actively voiding urine—ideally a few seconds after the dog starts but before it stops—what's referred to as a "a mid-stream sample." This is because samples collected at the very beginning of urination can sometimes collect debris in the urinary tract that is not associated with the bladder itself and contaminate the results, so a mid-stream sample is preferred.

Free catch samples are often valid when checking for other factors in the urine besides infection; for example, if you are looking for the presence of sugar or checking the dog's ability to concentrate its urine. For a specific test called the urine cortisol–creatinine ratio, a free catch sample collected at home is the **preferred** collection method as the stress of coming to the veterinary office can result in elevated cortisol levels that will adversely affect the test results.

The Cystocentesis Method

If your vet is trying to determine if your pet has a urinary tract infection, a free catch sample is not necessarily the best choice, mainly because the sample can get contaminated during the process of urination and give a false reading.

Urine in the bladder is supposed to be sterile: that means that there is not supposed to be any bacteria growing in the urine. But when the sample is collected with the free catch method, bacteria present in the urinary system further downstream from the bladder often contaminates the sample, or contamination occurs when urine passes through hair or across infected skin external to the urinary system. Sometimes dirt and other debris are also shed off the pet's coat into the sample. This can result in a false positive urine culture result, which can be very misleading when attempting to select the appropriate antibiotics.

The preferred method of urine collection when attempting to rule out a urinary tract infection (or to send urine for a culture and sensitivity) is by **cystocentesis.** During cystocentesis (also known as the "cysto"), the veterinarian will collect a urine sample through the body wall with a needle into a sterile syringe—this looks and sounds more appalling than it is!

Sometimes a small amount of blood can be introduced into a urine specimen this way, which can be misleading. Sometimes patient cooperation (or lack thereof) can force your veterinarian to opt for a different collection method. It is exceedingly difficult to obtain urine via cystocentesis on a dog who submissively wets for example! But these issues apart, the value of a cysto sample is that if there is evidence of infection in the sample, then you **know** that the infection is either at the level of the bladder or higher (meaning the kidneys could be involved).

Urinary Catheterization

Another, less commonly used method of collection is via urinary catheterization—another one not to try out at home! In this method, a urinary catheter is passed through the external opening, up the urethra, and into the bladder.

Catheterization is usually performed when a urinary obstruction is present (such as a bladder stone). It may also be performed to introduce a chemical dye (or sometimes air) into the bladder for the purposes of diagnostic radiographs ("x-rays").

A urine sample might be immediately collected through the catheter if it was used to relieve a urinary obstruction and the walls of the bladder are too damaged to sustain a needle puncture via cystocentesis.

Male dogs and cats are relatively easy to catheterize but are also far more likely to become physically obstructed by stones. Physical obstruction of the urinary system is a **life-threatening** situation and must be dealt with on an emergency basis. Female dogs are much harder to catheterize as the opening to the urethra is inside the vaginal vault and not easily identified. Female dogs may also develop bladder stones but can usually still urinate around them.

Urinary catheters can sometimes introduce infection into the bladder by nature of the fact that they are pushing up the urinary tract when normally urine flows in the reverse direction. If the open-ended catheters are left in place (that is urine if freely dripping out instead of into a closed container), then there is an open portal for infection into the urinary system because all the "gates" have been by-passed. For this reason, if a catheter must be left in place for an extended period, a closed collection system is usually preferred.

Section 5.2: The Components of Urinalysis

While your veterinarian will take note of such subjective findings such as color, odor, and clarity, it is the objective (or measurable) findings that are of most concern. While **urine specific gravity, the dipstick, and urine sediment** are the three main components, other tests are also useful.

Urine specific gravity (SPGR)

Specific gravity is another term for relative density: that is, ratio of the density of a substance (urine, in this case) to the density of a standard (plain water). The SPGR assesses the kidney's ability to concentrate urine, using a device called a refractometer to compare urine concentration to that of plain water. This will determine if the urine is being concentrated normally.

Think of it like this: water is taken in by the body and processed into urine. The kidneys must save a certain amount of water for running the body systems and eliminate the extra. Because the kidneys also eliminate certain bodily wastes into the urine, normal urine is usually more concentrated than water and has a higher specific gravity.

Urine specific gravity is subject to change however, dependent on how much water has been consumed that day (the more water you drink, the more diluted the urine) and how many waste products are present (the more the waste, the more concentrated the urine). A refractometer is an accurate means of measuring SPGR but can show a false increase in SPGR if the protein content of the urine is high or if certain dyes (contrast media for diagnostic radiographs) have been introduced into the urinary system.

The specific gravity of water is 1.000.

Normal urine concentration of dogs is between 1.030 and 1.040
(referred to as ten-thirty or ten-forty for the ease of saying it aloud).

Low SPGR Finding

A single finding of a specific gravity concentration less than ten-thirty does not necessarily indicate a problem, but **persistently low** specific gravities can indicate a problem with kidney function or the possibility of a metabolic problem resulting in the consumption of too much water.

A SPGR of 1.020 is considered "concentrating" but not fully. A follow up SPGR should be measured to see if the urine can concentrate higher than this, particularly if there are indications on the chemistry profile that kidney function is becoming less than ideal.

If a SPGR of 1.008 to 1.010 is so close to the SPGR of water, then the urine concentration is considered to be the same as water or **isosthenuric.** The water your pet drinks is coming out at the same rate it goes in without the body saving any for itself. Urine can be this dilute for many reasons, including disorders resulting in over-consumption of water, kidney disease, and Cushing's disease. A complete blood chemistry profile should be performed on any dog that is persistently isosthenuric.

Your veterinarian may also wish to run a **water deprivation test** to determine if your dog can concentrate the urine in the face of decreased intake. You must **never** attempt to run a water deprivation test yourself at home. In a controlled setting, your veterinarian will deprive your dog of water while measuring serial samples of urine for volume and concentration. At the same time, your dog will be closely monitored for signs of dehydration. At the first sign that your dog is becoming dehydrated in the face of water restriction, the test should stop, as this development indicates an inability to concentrate urine normally. This can help rule out dogs whose primary problem is a psychological over-consumption of water verses a dog that cannot concentrate urine because of a lack of antidiuretic hormone (ADH), as in the condition known as **diabetes insipidus** ("water diabetes"). Lack of concentrating ability due to other causes will usually have some supporting indication of the reason on the chemistry panel.

Your veterinarian may also ask you to measure your dog's water consumption over 24-48 hours to determine if your dog is drinking an excessive amount of water. **Normal volumes of water consumption for the dog are 20-90 ml/kg/day.**

Urine can be diluted to a SPGR even lower **(hyposthenuria)** by an active process of dilution by the kidneys. Although this number looks scary (1.005) it is indicative of some kidney function because the kidney must work to make the urine this dilute. Persistent hyposthenuria usually indicates resistance to or a lack of antidiuretic hormone (ADH). Lack of ADH is associated with diabetes insipidus (NOT the "sugar" diabetes—that's the diabetes mellitus we talked about in section 3.3). Resistance to ADH can be due to certain drug therapies, kidney infections, Cushing's disease, hypercalcemia, or amyloidosis.

Cats typically have urine concentrations 1.050 or higher unless they are on one of the urinary diets that increases water consumption. Very high urine concentrations can also be seen when an animal is dehydrated, although there are typically other signs of dehydration as well.

The Urine "Dipstick"

This is a plastic strip that has a series of chemical reagents attached to it. These reagents are designed to interact with various chemicals in the urine sample and undergo a color change that is then compared to a chart provided by the makers of the strips. The interpretation of these color changes is subjective and can be affected by the color of the urine itself, as well as operator error. A urine sample that is bright orange from an excess of bilirubin, for example, will tinge all the colored reagents with orange, making them less readily interpreted. Some newer urinalysis machines read the dipstick automatically, thus standardizing the results and removing the subjective assessment of different people.

After a urine sample is collected, it is spun in a centrifuge so that the cells and any debris will collect as **sediment** in the bottom of a centrifuge tube. The sediment is then examined separately. By taking this step prior to attempting dipstick analysis, sometimes you will get a more accurate sample for interpretation by dipstick. For example, a sample that is obviously discolored with blood may clear upon centrifugation to a yellow liquid component (called the **supernatant**) and the visible sediment. The supernatant can then be used for a more accurate dipstick analysis.

The dipstick usually contains anywhere from 8-10 components. The most common components are:

- urobilinogen

- bilirubin

- glucose

- ketones

- protein

- nitrite

- leukocytes

- blood

- pH

- specific gravity

NOTE: The measurement of SPGR by urine dipstick is often inaccurate and should not be relied upon when trying to determine if your dog is capable of concentrating urine. A refractometer is the preferred method of accurately assessing urine specific gravity, as we saw in the previous section.

We'll look now at each of these components of the dipstick.

Urobilinogen

Urobilinogen is a by-product of bilirubin production and metabolism. **Bilirubin** originates from aging red blood cells that are being stored in the liver and spleen. These red blood cells are broken down and then digested and converted into a form that is water-soluble (for excretion). Most bilirubin is converted into urobilinogen by the intestines and excreted through the feces—giving feces the bulk of its brown color. Small amounts are reabsorbed by the liver blood system (also known as the **portal** system) and excreted into the urine.

In theory, if there were a "back-up" somewhere in the system, the levels of urine urobilinogen would start to drop before other components of the bilirubin metabolism system, indicating early bile obstruction. The amount of urobilinogen would initially drop because the small amounts that are produced through the liver portal system would not be made or processed appropriately in the case of a bile duct obstruction. Later during obstruction, the inability to rid the body of excess bilirubin would result in excessive levels of bilirubin and its by-products in both the blood and urine. Unfortunately, urine urobilinogen cannot be relied upon to accurately identify liver problems due to its inherent instability. Often, no measurable amounts are detected in the urine of healthy dogs. Dogs on antibiotics or urinary acidifiers (vitamin C being a prime example) may also have decreased urine urobilinogen levels.

Excessive urobilinogen levels can occur when there is too much bilirubin in the system.

Think of it like this: only insignificant amounts of this product are made for excretion into the urine, and it is a fragile chemical product—easily altered by medications or supplements. So little to no urobilinogen can be normal. No urobilinogen could be abnormal, but that's hard to prove. Lots of urobilinogen means that there is something wrong with the bilirubin system, and the excess is being converted as best it can to urobilinogen. Chances are, however, that there will be more important markers at this point—such as the bilirubin levels themselves in the urine and blood.

Bottom line: this was a long section to explain why not much attention is paid to urine urobilinogen levels!

Urine Bilirubin

Urine bilirubin levels will rise before blood levels when there is an excess of bilirubin in the system. Once the body reaches the point where its capacity to excrete bilirubin is overcome, the levels will increase in the bloodstream as well.

When the bilirubin levels rise to 3-4 mg/dl in the bloodstream, the mucus membranes and visible skin will become noticeably yellow, and the dog is considered jaundiced or **icteric** (see discussion of bilirubin in section 3.2 of the chemistry profile). Thus, a dog with early autoimmune hemolytic anemia (AIHA) might first show increasing levels of bilirubin in the urine making it progressively darker orange in color. Then, as the anemic crisis continues, the serum will become visibly orange when the blood sample is centrifuged (which separates the blood into packed red cells and serum components). Finally, if unchecked, the AIHA will result in mucus membranes first being pale because of the anemia but becoming jaundiced as the bilirubin continues to rise.

A tumor obstructing the bile duct could also result in excessive bilirubin levels by preventing the normal cycle of excretion into the intestinal and urinary systems.

Note: It is possible to have significant liver disease and still have normal urine and blood levels of bilirubin, so as always, the different pieces of information (bloodwork, urinalysis, physical exam findings and clinical history) must be viewed in conjunction with each other.

Urine Glucose Levels

Urine Glucose levels should always be negative.

If the urine tests positive for glucose, then this usually indicates that more glucose is present in the bloodstream and higher levels are entering the kidneys to be eliminated into the urine.

High urine glucose levels can make the urine syrupy and sticky to the touch.

Persistently elevated urine glucose levels are usually indicative of diabetes mellitus (DM) – the condition discussed in section 3.3 when we looked at the chemistry profile values for the pancreas.

Tiny amounts of glucose will sometimes show up in urine temporarily (1-2 days) after a stressful event or a dose of steroids. Running a concurrent blood glucose level can help rule out this phenomenon. If the blood glucose levels are normal but there is a positive finding for glucose in the urine, this suggests a transitory event rather than persistent diabetes. Likewise, a slightly elevated blood glucose finding can be compared against the presence or absence of urine glucose to rule out excitability during the blood sample collection as a factor in the measured increase. Lack of a positive finding at that time would suggest that there is no significance to the slight elevation in the blood. Usually, a positive urine glucose test because of stress or steroids will be much less than that of a diabetic.

In certain rare kidney syndromes associated with defective absorption, the urine will also test positive for glucose. Marked bleeding into the urinary system can elevate urine glucose levels. But the first three potential causes for the persistent presence of glucose in the urine are 1. Diabetes mellitus. 2. Diabetes mellitus. 3. Diabetes mellitus.

Measuring the blood glucose or fructosamine levels can confirm or rule out such suspicions. There are many chemical agents and medications that can affect the results of a urine glucose test. It is important to collect a fresh urine sample for this test and avoid contamination with items such as bleach or hydrogen peroxide. If the urine sample is being examined primarily for the presence or absence of urine glucose (as opposed to examination for an infection) then the urine should not be refrigerated. Supplements such as vitamin C and antibiotics in the tetracycline family can falsely decrease urine glucose levels and make it difficult for the owner to monitor their degree of glucose regulation at home. There are certain drugs that have the potential to cause kidney damage. Often the urine glucose levels will elevate before evidence of kidney dysfunction is apparent on the blood chemistry panel.

A rare syndrome seen in certain breeds (such as the Basenji) called Fanconi syndrome can result in elevated urine glucose levels despite normal blood glucose levels (it is usually associated with concurrent elevations of blood phosphorus levels). Back in 2007, when tainted wheat gluten found its way into many assorted brands of pet food, some animals ended up with Fanconi-like syndromes due to the kidney damage. Tainted products continue to be an issue from time to time, and one of the biggest offenders is chicken jerky. I once spoke with a nutritionist from one of the major dog food companies, and she said she would never feed commercial chicken jerky to her own dog.

When in doubt, evaluate all the available lab work to determine the true cause of the glucosuria.

Ketones

The urine of dogs should be negative for ketones.

Ketones are the chemical by-products of excessive fat metabolism. They can occur during starvation when an animal is deprived of calories to the point that they are dissolving their fat stores at an excessive rate. Human diets (such as the Atkins diet or the popular keto diets) that restrict carbohydrates will also result in the formation of ketone bodies in the urine and blood. Pregnancy toxemia of women (and ewes) is an example of a metabolic condition that results in the formation of ketones.

The most usual form of **ketosis** in dogs is secondary to diabetes mellitus. DM places the dog in a catabolic state, where the rapid dissolution of fat stores acts in effect like a starvation diet. Ketosis is not desirable as a long-term metabolic state and can be life-threatening in some cases.

Note that ketones will show up in the urine (ketonuria) before the blood levels start to register them. If you have ketonuria, then DM must be ruled out. The presence of hyperglycemia (elevated blood glucose levels) plus ketonuria indicates a serious condition called **diabetic ketoacidosis**. This is an emergency condition that needs to be treated aggressively through hospitalization, fluid therapy, and insulin management until the ketoacidosis (and underlying diabetic state) is controlled. Ketonuria can also occur in aspirin overdoses. The highest levels of ketonuria are associated with diabetes, however.

Urine Protein Levels

Urine Protein levels are normally present in only trace amounts. The kidneys have an effective filtration system (the **glomerulus)** that is designed to keep the larger proteins from leaving the bloodstream and being excreted into the urine. Damage to the glomerulus apparatus will result in "holes" in the filtration device that will allow proteins to leak into the urine (proteinuria). The most common form of kidney dysfunction is **glomerular nephritis**, which is a progressive destruction of the glomeruli. It is important to remember that red and white cells are also made up of protein, so a urinary tract infection can result in elevated protein levels in the urine as well.

The test pad on the urine dipstick gives a range of color changes which, like glucose, correspond to the magnitude of the protein levels. It is important to take into consideration the SPGR when determining whether the protein levels are significant. In very dilute urine, even moderate levels of urine protein may be significant. Dogs with myelomas typically lose enormous quantities of protein into the urine but as these are what are termed "light-chain" proteins, then the dipstick is not valid for measuring this kind of protein loss (a separate test needs to be performed on dogs with suspected myeloma).

There are many potential causes of false readings on a dipstick analysis for protein, which is why your veterinarian may suggest an alternate form of testing if there are concerns about the protein levels in the urine. There are also many different medications and therapies that may result in secondary effects on the glomerulus, resulting in protein loss into the urine. First, one must decide if the level of protein in the urine is significant. Then all the potential medications and supplements that the dog might be taking should be evaluated as to potential effects. If a dog is taking medications that are known to have potential kidney-damaging effects (**nephrotoxic**), then these drugs should be stopped immediately until the cause of the proteinuria can be identified.

If the proteinuria is persistent and a urinary tract infection or inflammation has been ruled out, then the underlying cause is probably glomerular nephritis or amyloidosis. Amyloidosis is a condition where the normal filtration mechanism of the kidneys is gradually replaced by an abnormal protein that eventually replaces all the kidney tissue (think *Invasion of the Body-Snatchers!*). Glomerular nephritis is a progressive condition whereby something that causes chronic inflammation is punching holes in the glomeruli. Every attempt should be made to search for an underlying cause of the glomerular nephritis because the body cannot make new glomeruli. Heartworm disease, various tick-borne diseases such as Ehrlichia or Lyme, anything that can cause chronic inflammation such as long-standing cases of mange, pyometra, dental disease, and other chronic inflammatory diseases, such as lupus erythematosus, can result in glomerular nephritis. Just imagine a body having to constantly filter out junk because of chronic issues. That is going to increase the odds of developing glomerular nephritis. A kidney biopsy may be the only way to determine what the underlying cause is in some cases. There are certain breeds of dogs that are prone to hereditary glomerular nephritis as well.

Nitrites

Nitrites are included on most commercial urine dipsticks. In humans, the presence of nitrites in the urine increases if there are significant levels of bacteria in the urine. This does not seem to be as sensitive a test in dogs, but if the dipstick is positive for nitrites, then a urinary tract infection should be ruled out.

Leukocytes

Leukocytes (white blood cells) are also part of most urine dipsticks, but the urine should really be evaluated through a microscopic examination of the sediment to determine if leukocytes are present, as there are many artifacts that can alter the dipstick results. The presence of greater than

3-5 leukocytes per high power field on the microscope is considered significant. A "**high-powered field**" is the view through the eyepiece of the microscope on one of the higher settings, without moving the slide. So, if you are looking through the eyepiece of a microscope on 40 X (the strength of magnification), and you identify more than 3-5 leukocytes, then **pyuria** (pus in the urine) needs to be ruled out. A urinary tract infection is the most common cause of pyuria.

Blood

Blood in the urine is usually a significant finding. Trace amounts of blood may result in a urine sample collected by cystocentesis, but the other advantages in collecting a sterile sample by this method usually outweigh this negligible amount of contamination. Sometimes visually normal urine will test positive for blood on dipstick. This is because blood proteins will also react on the dipstick. In dogs, the most common cause of blood in the urine **(hematuria)** is a urinary tract infection. Hematuria can also result from tumors in the bladder, stones, and less commonly from kidney or prostatic disease (seen in older, intact male dogs) and from diseases such as leptospirosis. Frequently, bloody urine is seen with bleeding disorders. If your pet has blood in the urine, better make sure that they do not also have pale mucus membranes, which could indicate concurrent anemia as well.

Urine pH

Normally between 5-7 on a pH test strip

(With 7 being neutral).

The term pH stands for "potential of hydrogen" and is a scale that indicates the acidity or alkalinity of a liquid, usually urine or blood. Note: Chemical disinfectants contaminating the sample, as well as supplements such as methionine or vitamin C, can alter urine pH.

The urine pH can be affected by diet: carnivores tend to have a lower (or more acidic) pH while herbivores tend to have a higher (or more alkaline) urine pH.

Increased levels of urine pH are usually associated with a urinary tract infection in the dog. Abnormal urine pH levels also allow certain salts and minerals to precipitate out, or form crystals, in the altered urinary environment. Crystals can be extremely irritating and can lead to increased levels of red and white cells in the urine sediment (more on sediment later) as well as the formation of stones within the urinary system. When the urine pH returns to normal, these crystals will often disappear. There are many different types of crystals and stones that can form in urine under a wide variety of conditions. Determining the exact nature of the underlying problem is critical to finding a treatment solution.

Sometimes, the dog's own metabolism processes and excretes the minerals abnormally. Sometimes cheaper commercial dog foods do not get the balance of salts and minerals right, resulting in elevated urine pH and development of crystals. Special prescription diets are often recommended to control the precipitation of urinary crystals and prevent stone development. Because certain crystals form at certain pH levels, these special prescription diets have been formulated to keep your dog's urine pH within a certain range, depending on what the predominant crystal form has been.

In cats, the development of crystals in the urine is often associated with feeding dry cat food. Some brands are worse than others for creating crystals. While cats of both sexes can form crystals in their urine, the male cat's plumbing system means it's possible for the crystals to completely plug up the urethra. This is a life-threatening condition and requires emergency treatment. Many of these cats must eat special diets the remainder of their lives to prevent recurrence.

Unlike dogs, cats are prone to a syndrome that goes by many names: feline urological syndrome, feline lower urinary tract disease, feline interstitial cystitis, and more recently, pandora syndrome. It is believed that chronic anxiety and stress, with the anticipation of always being in a flight or fight response situation, is a major factor in why some cats develop chronic cystitis. As a side note, when the cat population within a single household reaches ten cats, there is a 100% probability someone will begin inappropriately urinating, so social interaction and hostility is probably a big factor in why some cats battle with urinary disease. So, keep in mind that diet may not be the only change your veterinarian recommends if your cat has this issue.

It is important not to supplement any animal on a special diet with urinary acidifiers such as methionine or vitamin C. If the animal is already on a urinary acidifying diet, the supplement may drive the urine pH too low (and potentially cause a new and different type of stone development). Added acidification may also negate the benefits to an animal on a urine neutral diet.

It is also important to remember that the predisposition to develop urinary crystals and stones can change over time and with aging. For example, Shih Tzus are prone to the development of struvite stones in early to middle age, and as such, may need a urinary acidifying diet. As the Shih Tzu ages, however, it becomes more prone to calcium oxalate stone formation, *which develops in acidic urine*. The **important** lesson here is to remember that just because your dog is prescribed a prescription diet to control a specific issue, do not assume that it is for life. You will need to have regular urinalysis tests performed to determine whether your dog should still be eating a specific prescription food. Some prescription foods can even be detrimental if fed into advanced senior status and you should be prepared to work with your veterinarian to alter your dog's diet over time as conditions change.

Note: Many of the newer urinary diets today are pH balanced to prevent both struvite crystals (which form in alkaline urine) and oxalate stones (which form in acidic urine). You may notice the designation S/O on the bag.

Other prescription foods, while quite necessary to prevent a life-threatening urinary blockage with stone formation, can be deficient in certain amino acids and may require special monitoring and supplementation. For example, male Dalmatians on a special diet to prevent ammonium urate stones may need to be supplemented with carnitine because of a hereditary predisposition to developing heart problems on this diet. In addition to regular urine checks to make sure the urine is being maintained at the correct urine pH for stone prevention, it is also recommended that these Dalmatians also have an echocardiogram every six months.

Urine Sediment Testing

Urine Sediment is created by centrifuging a urine sample so that any cells or crystals present within will collect in the bottom of the centrifuge tube in a form known as the **pellet**. By concentrating all the urine debris in this fashion, it is possible to examine it under the microscope for significant findings.

Urine that appears visually normal to the naked eye can have significant numbers of blood cells, white cells, or bacteria present. In addition to red blood cells, white blood cells, bacteria, and crystals, the technician will also be looking for the presence of epithelial cells that normally line the urinary system, as well as any abnormal cells or cells in abnormal numbers.

For instance, the presence of large numbers of transitional cells, which is a normal cell of the bladder lining, might indicate a transitional cell carcinoma (a bladder tumor). The tech will also look for **casts,** which are a conglomeration of mucoproteins that are formed by the distal tubules of the kidneys. (Think of them as little snakeskins—a technician can determine by cast identification what type of "snake" recently passed by—and potentially shed further light on kidney problems). The tech will also identify any crystals that may be present and look for bacteria too. Sometimes, it is possible to determine whether the bacteria identified are rods or cocci (the two most common categories), which can give your vet a head start as to determine the best antibiotic to use.

While extremely useful, sediment does not always tell the whole picture. It is possible to have stones present with absolutely normal urine sediment. No urinalysis can be considered complete without microscopic examination of urine sediment, however. Once a problem has been identified, your vet may not need to do a complete urinalysis each time he or she wants to screen for a specific issue. Your vet may only need to periodically check urine specific gravity or pH from time to time to monitor your dog's urinary situation.

Early Detection of Renal Dysfunction

This newer urine-screening test is gaining attention as a valuable tool in the early detection of kidney dysfunction. An in-house screening test, it examines your dog's urine for trace amounts of albumin. If you recall from section 3.5 on the blood chemistry values, albumin is a large protein—too large to be excreted by normal kidney glomeruli. Trace amounts in the urine is called **microalbuminuria.** This test can detect trace amounts of albumin in the urine long before the kidney dysfunction is severe enough to result in changes in BUN and creatinine on the blood chemistry panel.

Through such early detection means, some forms of kidney dysfunction can be addressed before significant destruction of the **nephrons** (the working unit of the kidney) has occurred. For the test results to be valid, however, you must be certain that no bladder infection is present, as an infection will falsely increase the protein levels in the urine. Some veterinarians are incorporating such tests into an overall-screening program for senior-aged dogs in order to identify problems at a point where intervention may still be useful.

NEWSFLASH

If you have one of the high-risk breeds for early development of kidney disease, you might want to consider screening for microalbuminuria using this test as a screening device during your dog's annual examination.

Urine Cultures

Urine cultures are used to identify the bacteria present in a suspicious urine sample and what types of antibiotics it may be sensitive to—therefore we often refer to a C & S or a culture and sensitivity. Urine cultures are not always necessary on a first time, uncomplicated urinary tract infection. If there are complicating factors (such as crystals) or there's a lack of response to the first chosen antibiotic, then your vet may suggest a C & S as the next step in addressing the problem. Certainly, if repeated infections occur, a C & S is recommended.

In most cases, the preferred method of collection for a C & S is by cystocentesis. Normal urine in the bladder is sterile. As we noted in section 5.1, by using a sterile collection method like cysto, if bacteria grow on the urine culture, then the source of the bacteria can be presumed to come from the level of the bladder or higher. If you submit a free-catch urine sample, there is the potential for contamination at several distinct levels—lower down in the tract, on the fur just outside the body, and so forth. That is not to say it's never appropriate to culture a free catch sample, just that these results must be viewed with this in mind. If a potentially contaminated sample is cultured and several different organisms grow colonies, sometimes there will be one predominant strain that is usually considered the significant organism causing the infection.

When urine is cultured at an outside laboratory, the sample is first incubated in a growth medium to maximize the potential for bacterial development. The growth medium/sample combination is then placed on several petri dishes filled with a gel that contains "bacteria food" called agar. Once the bacteria form colonies of growth on the agar plates, a series of tests allow the technician to precisely identify the type of bacteria present. Next, the laboratory technician will then transfer the concentrated sample onto agar plates that contain a series of disks that are impregnated with different antibiotics. A "zone of inhibition" will occur around any disk that contains an antibiotic that inhibits bacterial growth. The size of the zone indicates whether the bacteria are sensitive, insensitive, or resistant to the effects of the specific antibiotic. Some human laboratories will use very new and expensive antibiotics in their selection of drugs to test sensitivity, which are not always practical for veterinary use, so it is best to use a veterinarian-based lab if possible.

Once it has been determined bacteria are present in the sample and which antibiotics are effective against the bacteria, your vet will decide which is the most appropriate antibiotic to use. Your vet must weight factors such as cost, effectiveness, and potential side effects when choosing the appropriate medication. An effective, inexpensive medication is of no use if 50% of the animals taking are likely to vomit. Alternatively, if we reach for the "big guns" every time we dispense a medication, we are in danger of fostering the further development of antibiotic resistance. It is a very real concern that common organisms such as streptococcus and staphylococcus have become resistant to so many of our antibiotics. There are people in the medical community who predict that sometime in the not-too-distant future, the failure to find an effective antibiotic for some of these common organisms will be the biggest threat to public safety that we face.

If your vet determines that a urine culture is in order, but your dog has already been on antibiotics, it may be necessary to allow several weeks to pass without any antibiotic therapy at all to prevent the possibility that, although not effective in eliminating the infection, the antibiotic being given was sufficient to suppress the bacterial growth to the point that you get a false negative culture result.

At the time of writing, there are some in-house test kits available that will allow your veterinarian to perform a limited urine culture in a shorter period than some of the outside laboratories. These kits will identify the presence of a few categories of bacteria (the most common ones seen in urinary tract infections) and the effectiveness of a few antibiotics (the most prescribed). These tests can be especially useful as a quick, less expensive screening method than a traditional C & S, but if the bacteria present are uncommon, you may end up with false negative results.

Urine Cortisol–Creatinine Ratios

The ratio of the two values should be less than 20

Cortisol–creatinine ratios are measured by collecting a urine sample in a non-stressful manner (usually caught by the owner at home) and measuring the values of these substances that are excreted into the urine.

The ratio of these numbers is beneficial primarily when you are suspicious of the possibility of Cushing's disease or **hyperadrenocorticism** (a condition in which the body is producing elevated levels of cortisol due to a tumor secreting a particular hormone). The excess cortisol spills over into the urine for excretion from the body. Because creatinine levels have a direct correlation to glomerular filtration rate, comparing the ratio between the two substances can help rule in or rule out Cushing's disease. A dog with normal cortisol–creatinine ratios **cannot** have Cushing's. This is a useful screening test. It is less expensive than the test usually used to examine for Cushing's (either the "ACTH stim" test or the low-dose dexamethasone), and if your dog falls into the small margin of dogs where the ACTH stim test is ambiguous, it can help clarify the results. Of course, if the results are abnormal, then an ACTH stim test is warranted (more on that test in Section 11).

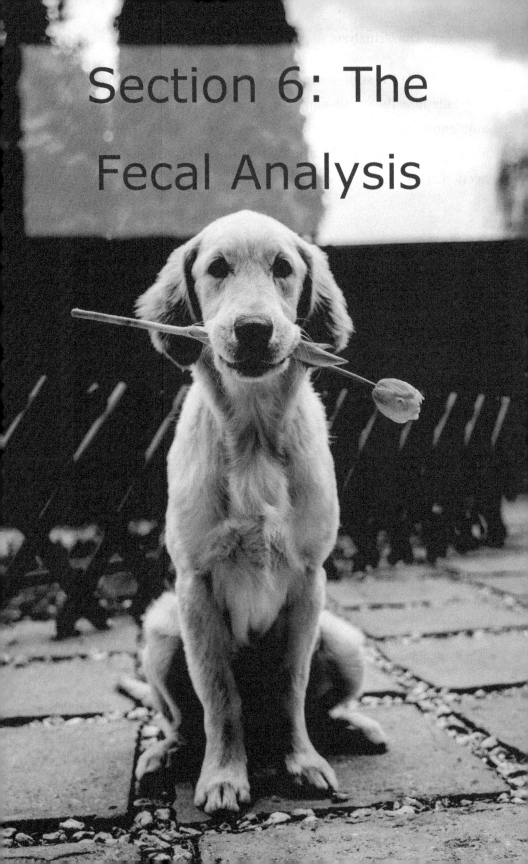

Section 6: The

Fecal Analysis

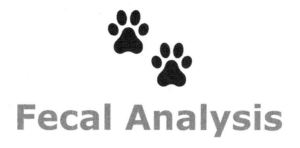

Fecal Analysis

One might be under the impression that there was only so much information that could be gathered from studying feces. After all, your dog either has worms or it doesn't, right? But fecal analysis tells us much more, and there is a lot of information to be gathered from examining how your pet processes his or her food. It's wise to bring a fresh stool sample with you every time you take your dog to the vet's office. If the sample is not needed, then the staff can dispose of it for you.

Section 6.1: What Does It Look Like?

Let's start with appearance. The quality of the poop is influenced strongly by diet. Dogs that eat a balanced home-cooked diet or on the BARF diet (Bones and Raw Foods, for those unfamiliar with the term) are usually going to have smaller, more compact stools than dogs that eat commercial kibble (dry dog food). Stools vary widely with types of kibble as well, with some diets resulting in soft, less compact stools that are produced four-six times daily. More typical are firm brown stools produced 2-3 times daily. Highly colored food usually results in stools of a similar color.

If you have been feeding your dog the same food for a while, you should be familiar with the normal appearance of his poop. Changes in appearance can be significant.

Stools that become black and sticky like tar can be indicative of bleeding into the gastrointestinal (GI) tract. **Melena** is digested blood, which means that the bleeding is coming from higher up in the GI tract, such as in the stomach or small intestines. Ulcers secondary to the use of non-steroidal anti-inflammatories (NSAIDs) or steroid therapy are the most common cause of melena in the dog. Melena can also result from bleeding tumors high in the GI tract. Melena is a serious condition and warrants immediate contact of your veterinarian.

Administration of Pepto Bismol to your pet can also cause a marked darkening of the stool. The stool can be anywhere from clay colored to black on Pepto Bismol. Clay-colored stools can also indicate a bile obstruction, as most of the stool color comes from the secretion of bile into the intestines. Be sure to let your vet know if you have administered any over-the-counter medications when you discuss abnormal stool appearance. Pepto Bismol (and now the "new and improved" Kao pectate as well) contains small amounts of subsalicylate, which is related to aspirin. You should not administer these products without consulting your veterinarian, as it may react negatively with other medications or be contraindicated in a bleeding disorder.

Blood that is fresh or bright red is referred to as "frank" blood when present in the stool. This indicates blood from a source lower in the intestinal tract, usually the colon. Inflammation of the colon may result in **colitis,** in which your dog may strain to produce scant amounts of a loose stool with frank blood and mucus. While it looks alarming, most dogs do not appear to feel bad with colitis. However, colitis must be distinguished from **hemorrhagic gastroenteritis**. HGE usually results in stool the consistency of strawberry jam and can be a life-threatening situation. Dogs with HGE are usually sicker than dogs with colitis and have evidence of **hemoconcentration** (excessively high PCV) on the CBC. HGE may require hospitalization and IV fluid therapy to treat, so when in doubt, see your veterinarian. HGE is more likely to affect small breeds of dogs, but in both colitis and HGE, the inappropriate consumption of a particular food item is usually the trigger.

Diarrhea

This is a general term to describe stool that is not formed normally. Diarrhea can be anything from explosive, watery stool in large volumes to small, scant, and gelatinous stools.

Veterinarians attempt to classify the type of diarrhea as to either large or small bowel diarrhea. If one can localize the problem to a particular section of the GI tract, then you can focus on the list of potential causes. The causes of large verses small bowel diarrhea are quite different, and it helps to know which type of problem you are dealing with. The descriptive nature of the diarrhea can convey a lot of information to your veterinarian. My four favorite descriptors are "watery," "pudding-like," "soft-serve ice cream" and "melted ice cream". My clients can easily form a mental picture of what each description looks like and can relay the necessary information accordingly.

Small Bowel Diarrhea

Small bowel diarrhea is usually explosive, watery, and there's a lot of it. Dogs typically feel unwell in the acute form; there may or may not be concurrent vomiting. If the diarrhea is more chronic, these dogs usually lose weight. Dehydration can be of major concern.

Small bowel diarrhea often results from "trash-canitis" (or some such inappropriate consumption of an item that may or may not be food) and is not typically a chronic problem. It will often change into large bowel diarrhea as it begins to resolve.

Chronic small bowel diarrhea is indicative of fundamental problem with the food processing mechanism. It can result from a cellular infiltrate (as in inflammatory bowel disease or cancer) that is making the bowel walls too thick to absorb nutrients or indicate a maldigestion-malabsorption syndrome such as pancreatic exocrine insufficiency (PEI). It can also be an indication of a food allergy.

In any case, chronic small bowel diarrhea may require an extensive work-up to get to the root of the problem, including radiographs, food trials, maldigestion profiles, endoscopy with biopsy, or an ultrasound.

Large Bowel Diarrhea

This is usually scant in volume. Dog may strain (the act of which is called **tenesmus**) to produce small "gloppy" stools. There may or may not be frank blood or mucus. The straining, as well as the presence of blood, may look as though your dog is constipated. Dogs **rarely** get truly constipated. Dogs have the capacity to ingest and pass the most incredible substances. In cases when dogs ingest something that they cannot pass, they usually stop eating and are incapable of keeping even water down without vomiting. In most cases, straining to defecate in dogs is associated with large bowel diarrhea instead of an impaction.

Cats, on the other hand, can develop megacolon (a baggy, flaccid colon incapable of evacuating stools) that can result in a condition called **obstipation**. Your cat will need medical intervention to treat this condition, which may include enemas. However, under no circumstances should you attempt to give an enema to your pet at home! Many human enemas contain ingredients that are lethal to pets, and a damaged colon can rupture if not treated appropriately. Straining to defecate or not defecating regularly is grounds for having your pet examined by your veterinarian.

Colitis is large bowel diarrhea in the acute form. If it is a chronic problem, the list of things that can result in large bowel diarrhea are much shorter than the causes of small bowel diarrhea, with food intolerances or parasites heading the list. Dogs with large bowel diarrhea typically have normal appetites and do not usually lose significant amounts of weight.

Section 6.2: The Fecal "Float"

A test for parasites, the float, consists of a variable amount of fresh poop collected from your pet and suspended in a supersaturated salt or sugar solution. The supersaturated solution will allow the lighter parasite eggs to separate from the fecal material and rise to the surface of the solution. (The concentration of salt in the Dead Sea is so high that it is virtually impossible for a person to sink in it—same concept here).

The presence of parasite eggs will be detected when they float to the top of the solution and stick to a thin piece of glass called a coverslip, which is then transferred to a microscope slide and examined. As a quick screening tool in the veterinary hospital, this test is about 80% effective in identifying the presence of parasite eggs. You may be asked to provide more than one fecal sample to rule in or out a particular problem.

It is possible to miss the presence of parasites in sparse numbers. Whipworms, which live in the large bowel, often fail to show up on a routine fecal analysis yet can still be present in significant numbers. This is because eggs are not always shed continuously in stool, and some samples can be void of any eggs at all. Using a large volume of stool for analysis (as much as two grams) and then centrifuging it to concentrate potential egg numbers, much as you do with urine sediment, can improve accuracy. Some parasites, most notably **Giardia**, will be destroyed by the standard salt solution and can only be identified if special solutions are used. Tapeworms shed their eggs in segmented sections of their bodies, which break off and are excreted with the feces. Because the eggs are inside the segments, they may not show up on a fecal analysis. This is why your veterinarian may opt for a **therapeutic trial** of a dewormer in the absence of any positive egg findings.

A wet mount or direct smear is used when trying to identify certain motile (moving) organisms or bacteria. A single drop of fresh feces is mixed with normal saline and examined under the microscope at a higher power than the microscope strength typically used to examine feces. The saline solution is not supersaturated, so the organisms can continue to swim about on the slide (making them much easier to identify). Sometimes this test is used as a "quick and dirty" screening for Giardia, as the trophozoites are easily spotted while swimming.

Because we are starting to see parasite resistance to our standard medications and because mutations are happening with greater frequency, there is concern that the floatation methods may miss significant number of parasites or misidentify the parasites themselves. There is also concern, given the development of certain strains of parasites that have developed resistance, that we may not be utilizing deworming agents wisely. Some veterinary clinics are moving away from in-house testing by the floatation method and sending samples to outside laboratories for more specific **fecal antigen testing**, which is highly accurate but more expensive and takes longer to get results. These specialized tests may become more common as we struggle to deal with parasite resistance, as these tests can detect a wide range of parasites in one sample, as well as determine if they pose a threat to both pets and their owners.

Sometimes, special stains are used to identify certain bacterial organisms. Your vet may also wish to perform **rectal cytology** in the process of working up a case of chronic diarrhea. A sample of rectal mucosa is collected via scraping the surface of it with a swab and rolling it out on the surface of a microscope slide. The presence of inflammatory cells or certain types of bacteria may help pinpoint the cause of a chronic problem. Sometimes your vet may wish to perform a **fecal culture** if there is concern that a particular bacterial type is causing illness in your dog. A sample of feces is then sent to an outside laboratory where the lab will attempt to "grow" bacteria within the sample on petri dishes and then determine through various tests what type of bacteria it is. Of course, there are many, many bacteria present in feces, but if an overwhelming number of a particular type is present, and that type is known to cause disease, then you can be certain that the results are significant.

Section 6.3: Parasites of the Dog

Briefly, let us discuss the most common parasites of the dog found in a fecal sample. (I just know some of you have microscopes sitting at home that you are dying to use!) Even if you are not a budding parasitologist with your own mini lab at home, there are some basic facts about the life cycle and transmission of worms that are good to review.

Parasites can have a serious health impact on both young and adult dogs. I once watched a continuing education session about anemia in dogs and had to shake my head at the instructor's bland assumption that parasites need not be on a list of potential causes when working up a case of anemia in an adult dog. Maybe not in some other parts of the country, but in the Mid-Atlantic region where I live and work, it is possible to see flea and parasite infestations **kill** adult large breed dogs.

Pet owners can't afford to take parasites lightly.

Roundworms

Roundworms are the most common parasite seen in puppies. Worms are sneaky creatures. They are so co-dependent with their host species that they can maximize their success moving into the next host in interesting and unsuspected ways. Roundworms are a fine example of this.

When a young dog gets roundworms, a natural resistance starts to develop at around 3 months of age. (Note: the resistance does not confer immunity, just lessens the degree of impact the worm has upon its host). This resistance causes some worms to become dormant in the muscle tissues in an immature form. In a male dog (or a spayed female), this is a dead-end cycle. In the breeding bitch, however, as the milk production begins to come into gear, the dormant worms wake up and migrate into the milk glands where (TA-DA!) they are consumed by the nursing puppies. Roundworms can also cross the placenta directly and infect puppies before birth. At four weeks of age, some puppies can already have life-threatening numbers of intestinal worms.

As few as one hundred roundworms can kill a puppy, usually through intestinal blockage. The only way to break this cycle is to deworm the bitch with a fenbendazole-type dewormer during the last five days of pregnancy. Easier and safer is using a pyrantel-type dewormer on all puppies at four weeks of age and again at six weeks, but pyrantel is one of the products we're seeing become less effective as a dewormer. Bottom line, talk to your vet about the best products available. The local feed store or pet store may not be the best place to get your deworming agents, in part because of parasite resistance.

Adult dogs get infected when your dog accidentally swallows roundworm eggs from the soil (by licking feet...etc.). Once ingested, the immature worms migrate through the liver and lungs and then back to the intestines where they mature into egg-laying adults. These eggs are then passed with the poop into the soil. It takes about three weeks for the eggs to become infective to the next host, so if you have dogs in pens, regular poop scooping can help decrease the numbers of eggs present in the environment. Heavy infections can result in damage to the liver, lungs, and even the brain. Roundworms can sometimes infect people through hand-mouth contact with contaminated soil.

Larval migrans is a term used to describe the abnormal migration of worm larvae through tissue, especially in humans who are exposed to dog or cat roundworms. The worms do not know how to act in an atypical host! When roundworms migrate across the retina, the result can be permanent vision damage or blindness.

Puppies with "rounds" typically have a pot-bellied, unhealthy look. Vomiting and diarrhea are not uncommon, but it is also possible not to have any obvious signs at all. Sometimes pups will pass volumes of roundworms in the stool or vomit them up. The adult worms resemble long strands of spaghetti when voided in this fashion. The nickname "roundworms" may have evolved to distinguish the appearance of these worms from the "flatworms," such as tapeworms (the other most observed worm by you, the client).

Under the microscope, roundworm eggs have often been described as looking like a "hamburger on a plate," as seen from the top view, looking down from above.

Hookworms

These are the bad boys of the parasite world. They are blood-feeders, with little hook-like attachment spikes in their mouths that allow them to burrow their mouth parts into the intestinal wall. They secrete an anti-coagulant so that as they feed, there is no shortage of blood flow.

Severe hookworm infestations can result in life-threatening anemia in both puppies and adult dogs. The cumulative effect of the anticoagulant from many worms can cause mildly delayed clotting times. Again, the eggs are usually swallowed by the animal, but they can also be picked up through the skin by sitting on a patch of damp, sandy soil (in humans this causes a fierce skin rash). Hookworms can also be transferred across the placenta before the puppies or kittens are born and through the mother's milk.

Because the life cycle of the hookworm takes only two weeks from ingestion of an egg to the production of mature egg-laying adults, it can be exceedingly difficult to control infestations on your property without the regular use of products to control hookworms. Unless you are prepared to deworm your dogs every two weeks, once you get hookworms on your property it is usually necessary to use a heartworm preventative that also is effective against "hooks" to prevent serious complications of infection. You might never see hookworms being passed in the stool, so the absence of diarrhea or visible worms in the stool does not rule out the presence of serious parasites! Not all over the counter dewormers will be effective against hookworms, so read your labels before assuming your product is effective. Better yet, talk to your veterinarian. Hookworm resistance to common dewormers is a very real problem in some areas.

Under the microscope, hookworm eggs are more oval than round and appear as a thin-walled oval sac with a series of round balls contained within.

Whipworms

Whipworms live in the large intestine, and their eggs are not shed on a regular basis. Known as a "whipworm" because one end is thickened like a whip handle, and the remainder of the worm stretches out into a thin cable, much like a bullwhip. They are a common cause of large bowel diarrhea in the dog. It's often hard to prove they are present. The life cycle of the whipworm is exceptionally long with as much as 4-6 months between the time of infestation to the appearance of eggs in feces.

Whipworm eggs have thick walls and are resistant to disinfectants. A prescription dewormer is usually necessary to treat for "whips," as most over-the-counter products will not affect them. Severe infections can cause pronounced weight loss and diarrhea. Dogs living in outdoor pens previously infected with whipworm eggs can develop life-threatening infections.

Whipworms eggs appear like brown footballs with a bubble at each pointed end when viewed on the microscope slide. The "bubble" is a little trap door called an **operculum,** which opens as the egg matures into the next phase of development. There are very few operculated intestinal worm eggs, so this makes the whipworm egg quite easy to identify when it is present. The adult whipworm is rarely voided in the feces, so you are not likely to see them. Most people will never see a whipworm in the stool.

Whipworms are a common cause of severe diarrhea and weight loss. Because whipworms are sometimes hard to find on fecal analysis, they are one of the main reasons your vet may choose to do a therapeutic deworming in the absence of a positive fecal result. Very few over the counter dewormers will be effective against whips; a prescription product is usually necessary.

Tapeworms

Tapeworms are the most common intestinal parasite that you, the client, are likely to see. Tapeworms are flatworms, belonging to a different class of worms than the others already mentioned. Tapes appear as fresh segments either on your dog's feces or sometimes dried on the hair around the anus. This is because the tapeworm is a segmented flatworm that breaks off into small pieces as it passes out of the dog's body. People describe them as looking like pieces of rice or pumpkin seeds, depending on how dried out they are when they are noticed. The dog must eat an intermediate host to get a tapeworm infection. This is usually a flea but can also be a small rodent or rabbit. If your dog or cat has tapeworms, you should be looking for fleas!

Although these are unsightly parasites to see and despite the jokes about tapeworms making you lose weight, as parasites go, tapeworms seldom cause clinical illness. So, if you see tapeworm segments on your dog on a Saturday afternoon, then you should rule out fleas as the source but do not rush off in a panic to the ER. Your vet will want a fecal sample to rule out other worms as well. Very few over the counter dewormers will be effective against tapeworms; a prescription product is usually necessary. Tapeworm eggs will often NOT appear on a fecal analysis because the eggs are inside the segments and do not always get mixed into the poop but sit on the surface of it only. That is one reason is possible for your vet to report a "negative" fecal result, and then you spot a tapeworm segment days later.

Coccidia

Coccidia are not technically "worms" at all but protozoan parasites. Coccidia seldom cause clinical signs in an adult dog but in puppies can cause such severe bloody diarrhea and dehydration that can mimic parvo in the severity of clinical signs. Sometimes, the puppy can present with neurological signs (altered mentation, stupor...etc.) as well, if the oocysts have penetrated the nervous system. Coccidia is easily spread in the soil, and puppies housed in dirt pens outside will often have high numbers of oocysts.

This parasite is potentially infectious to humans as well. It takes 4-5 days from the time that an oocyst is passed in the feces to the time that it is infective to the next host, so cleaning up the poop in the area is important. Washing your hands after handling poop and/or the puppy is necessary during treatment.

A prescription medication specifically aimed at controlling coccidia is needed to clear infections. These medications do not kill the coccidia organism but prevent it from reproducing until all the oocysts die off. You will often have to treat a dog for 5-7 days with a coccidia medication.

The oocysts are exceedingly small when viewed under the microscope and can potentially be missed by a technician who is only scanning the fecal sample under a low (4X) power. They resemble an oval that is slightly more pointed at one end and contain 1-2 central nuclei that remind me of eggs sunny side up on a plate.

Giardia

Giardia is another protozoan parasite that must be treated with a prescription medication. It is usually picked up through drinking contaminated ground water.

Dogs are resistant to the effects of giardia. All the streams and ponds in my home state are considered to contain this parasite, yet we seldom see dogs that are truly ill from it. It can cause serious problems in small puppies or in weak, debilitated animals. As such, it should be considered in any case of chronic diarrhea. It is a hard parasite to identify. The typical salt solutions used to float worm eggs will dehydrate giardia trophozoites (these are the protozoa in their active, feeding stage of their life cycle). It is necessary to use a special solution to float these organisms for identification, and even then, your vet may have to run five consecutive daily samples to rule out the presence or absence of this parasite. It is often easier and less expensive to simply treat for giardia and see what the response to treatment might be.

The trophozoites attach to the intestinal wall cells and effectively block out their ability to absorb nutrients. The cell then ruptures, releasing more of the organisms that go on to attach to other cells.

Giardia can cause profound diarrhea and significant weight loss. Dogs with giardia often lose the ability to digest and absorb fat, so the diarrhea is often rancid in odor and fatty in appearance. Because this can mimic other maldigestion/malabsorption conditions, your vet may recommend a therapeutic trial on an anti-giardia medication as part of a work-up of chronic diarrhea. Trophozoites are **motile;** they are one of the few parasites that "swim" when viewed on a wet mount (the concentration of saline not being strong enough to dehydrate them in that method). It is always fun to peer into the microscope and see hundreds of little organisms propelling themselves around by swishing their flagella. When it happens, you can be very sure you are dealing with a case of giardia, and that is usually extremely rewarding to treat.

NEWSFLASH

Worms can kill. Deworm with appropriate products or have your vet help you design a program that will keep your dog healthy.

Fecal analysis will only identify intestinal parasites 80% of the time. When in doubt repeat the fecal or deworm anyway!

Assume puppies and kittens have worms until proven otherwise. Have your young pet dewormed at an early age and checked at least twice during their wellness exams.

It may be necessary for you to use a prescription heartworm preventative that helps control other parasites once the property has been seeded with parasite eggs.

Diarrhea does not necessarily equal worms. There are many causes of diarrhea and the appearance of the stool and description of how your dog passes a movement can help narrow the list of differential choices.

Section 7:

Heartworm Disease

Testing

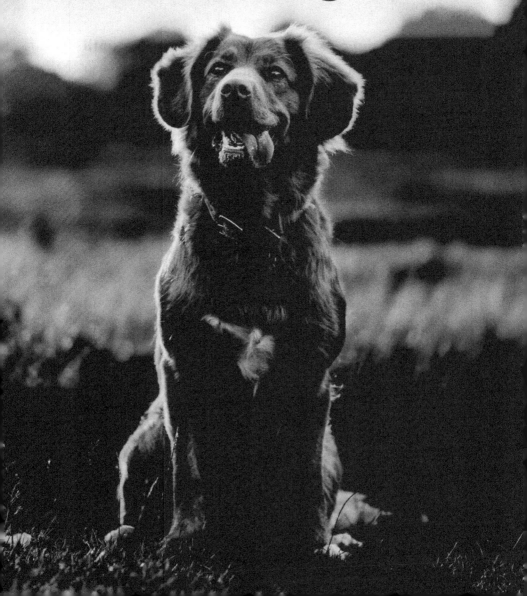

Heartworm Disease Testing

A recent study released by the American Heartworm Society states that only 55% of the dogs in the U.S. are currently taking heartworm preventative. If you look at the spread of heartworm disease since it first became widely reported in 1975, the results are frightening.

Mosquitoes transmit heartworms but don't think they're only a problem of the Deep South in the summertime. Just like West Nile Virus and certain tick-borne diseases, the heartworms have spread further north and west over the last 30 years until they are endemic (widespread) in nearly every state at this time. If you are relying on the fact that your neighbors are limiting the spread of heartworms by having their dogs on preventatives, and thus creating a zone of protection around your dog, you could be wrong. If you are thinking that your dog is an indoor dog and therefore is safe, you are also wrong (safer, yes; immune? No). And if you think that giving heartworm preventative on a regular basis is somehow less healthy than not doing so, it is important that you make yourself familiar with the effects of this devastating disease before you make this decision on behalf of your dog.

Being an informed pet owner means keeping an open mind, weighing the information gathered, and deciding based on the best information available at the time. Before choosing to alter your vaccine program, you should weigh the risks of local exposure to infectious disease against the possibilities of undesirable side effects of vaccines. You might choose to titer your dogs (see Section 12) rather than vaccinate annually or you may decide to vaccinate for fewer diseases. Before abandoning your vaccine protocol altogether, it would be wise to recall that in the early days of parvo, the disease raced through the dog population like wildfire until it was brought under control with vaccination. My first job out of school was in an extremely rural area where most people didn't vaccinate their pets. I saw forty cases of parvo the last month I worked at that practice. I saw entire litters succumb to this preventable disease. In this same area, seven out of ten dogs had heartworms. We treated on average seven dogs a week by injecting them with an arsenic-based product. Though heartworm treatment has improved since then, the disease is still fraught with significant risk and the potential for irreversible organ damage. Before deciding to discontinue heartworm preventative for your dog, you need to do a risk/benefit analysis.

Heartworm Life Cycle

Let's look at the life cycle of the heartworm. A mosquito bites a dog infected with heartworms. While having its meal (blood), the mosquito ingests **microfilaria** (the immature, microscopic form of heartworm). The microfilaria matures in the mouthparts of the mosquito into what is called the "L3" form. It is this L3 microfilaria that the mosquito deposits under the skin of the next dog it bites, infecting the dog with tiny immature heartworms.

The L3 form migrates from the fine capillaries of the skin into the deeper tissues through the bloodstream, and after 45 days, matures into the L4 stage. The immature stages of the heartworms continue to migrate, passing through most of the high blood volume organs, such as the lungs, liver, and kidneys, causing damage along the way. Four to six months after the initial infection by the mosquito, adult heartworms are now lodged in the right ventricle of the heart, obstructing blood flow and increasing the workload on the heart. At that time, circulating microfilaria may become apparent in the dog's bloodstream, and the infected dog serves as a reservoir for the next mosquito to come along. By this time, a dog will test positive for heartworms through the various testing methods available.

How Often Should You Test for Heartworm?

Because of the efficacy of the newer treatments, many practices adopted an every-other-year testing policy. If you live in an area where prevention is not needed year-round, you should seriously consider testing early each spring **before** re-starting prevention coverage. That's because **administration of a heartworm preventative to a dog with circulating microfilaria can result in anaphylaxis and sudden death.** If you are not giving heartworm preventative year-round, there is a window of exposure where your pet can be infected. Even if you are religiously administering a monthly heartworm preventative (never late, never skip a dose by mistake), regular testing is necessary.

There are also concerns that like other parasites, we may be starting to see resistance to heartworm preventatives too. You should discuss with your veterinarian the best products to use and how often to test. Many of the companies that make the most popular heartworm preventatives have product guarantees that will help pay for treatment should your dog get heartworms, but only if you have annual testing performed and you buy your products from a veterinarian (and not an online pharmacy, where counterfeit products can be an issue).

I once saw a nine-year-old Pit Bull that was dying of end-stage heartworm disease. He was in multi-system organ failure due to the advanced nature of his infection with the heart, lungs, liver, and kidneys all involved. It took quite a bit of persuading before the client would allow me to perform a heartworm test to confirm the diagnosis because the client was convinced that she had never missed a dose of preventative in the four years since the dog was last tested. What was so very discouraging in this case was had the dog been tested annually, the disease would have been identified in the early stages before the major damage had occurred, potentially resulting in successful treatment before it was too late.

Certain parasites and the diseases they cause can vary a great deal by region, even within the same state. A person in my immediate area who chooses not to use heartworm preventatives or titers their adult dogs instead of periodic vaccination is taking less of a risk than a person in a coastal or metropolitan area making the same choices. This is not only because of a greater incidence of disease in certain areas but due to **herd immunity** as well. If most pets in your area are well-vaccinated against common diseases, then it is harder for an outbreak to occur because there are fewer susceptible animals in the first place. It is also important to remember that things can change. When I first moved to my current location, we almost never saw Lyme or other tick diseases. Then deer ticks infiltrated our location, and the incidence of tick-borne disease shot through the roof. Currently, we see little heartworm disease, but every new subdivision is putting in a retaining pond to catch runoff, and our mosquito populations are on the rise. Decisions about vaccinations or parasite control need to be fluid as things change.

The Advantages Of "Snap" Tests

This is a good place to talk about the heartworm tests that also test for exposure to tick borne diseases such as Lyme, Anaplasmosis, and Ehrlichiosis, as well as the difference between **antigen** tests and **antibody** tests. When the so-called "snap" tests for heartworm disease detection were created, this proved to be a big boon to veterinarians looking for an inexpensive and uncomplicated way to test for heartworm disease in the clinic without having to send samples out for testing. Because these early heartworm tests were **antigen** tests, they could detect occult heartworm disease: disease in which there were no circulating microfilaria or in which there were very few adult worms. The tests are considered highly accurate because they are reacting to the presence of **antigens** created by the actual heartworms.

More recently, screening for other serious diseases have been added to these snap tests. In dogs, these snap tests now also screen for common tick-borne disease. In cats, heartworm testing is sometimes combined with feline leukemia and feline immunodeficiency testing. Some of these additional tests are not antigen tests like the heartworm portion but look for the presence of **antibodies** instead. Antibodies are made by the body in response to exposure to certain antigens, but antibodies do not necessarily equate with disease in the body—they indicate *exposure* to that disease. Most dogs who test positive for Lyme on a snap test don't necessarily have Lyme; they've been exposed at some point in the past and are making antibodies against it. Therefore, we frequently recommend additional testing to determine if this is merely an antibody reaction or a bona fide infection. So, why do we test at all if it's only an antibody test? Well, for one thing, if the tests are negative, you can take some of these potential diseases off the table. It's also a quick way of getting information on the spot instead of waiting on outside laboratory test results.

Why does your vet sometimes recommend treatment based on these test results, even if a positive result might only be an antibody reaction? It may depend on why your vet decided to run the tests in the first place. If your pet has certain symptoms, then treating for a positive antibody reaction may make sense instead of waiting days to weeks for other test results to come in.

But keep in mind when your dogs "tests positive for Lyme" this does NOT automatically mean he has Lyme. It simply means he tests positive. If he tests positive, has a fever, joint pain, and kidney issues, then Lyme should move to the top of the diagnostic list. If he has all these clinical signs but tests negative for Lyme, then you need to look for a different disease that will cause these symptoms.

See Section 8 for more information about Lyme Disease.

Heartworm Preventatives

Many of the heartworm preventatives can be used as part of an overall program to control other parasites in addition to heartworms. You may need to discuss with your veterinarian which heartworm preventative is the most appropriate for your pet. In areas that are heavily infested with heartworms and/or experience short, mild winters, it may be advisable to continue heartworm preventive year-round.

Again, this is best determined depending on your immediate area, the places you travel with your dog during the winter months, and the local incidence of heartworm disease. If you live in an area where it is possible to stop heartworm preventative during the winter months, it will be necessary to re-test your dog annually before re-starting the preventative, just in case break-through exposure has occurred and to avoid the risk of anaphylaxis. Dogs that are on year-round heartworm preventative are usually tested on an annual or every-other-year basis. If your life is hectic or if remembering to get in for testing at the right time of year is a problem (and be honest with yourself!), then year-round prevention may be the best way to go.

When heartworm disease was first recognized and preventatives developed, the daily preventative was the only option. At the time, veterinarians had to draw a significant sample of blood (usually 1-2 milliliters), treat it with a preservative, centrifuge it to concentrate the parasites in the sample, and examine the sample under the microscope for the presence of microfilaria. This method was 97% accurate in determining if heartworms were present because the available heartworm preventatives worked through preventing microfilaria from penetrating into the deeper tissues. Therefore, in the absence of microfilaria, the dog was considered heartworm negative. However, it could miss **occult** (silent) heartworm infections. If a dog was infected with only a single sex of heartworms (and therefore no microfilaria was produced) or had only a very few heartworms, it might be possible to miss any microfilaria in the sample. Also, because mosquitoes feed at night, microfilaria numbers could wax and wane during the day. I once had a patient that tested heartworm negative by this method at 9 a.m. and positive at 5 p.m. on the same day...

In addition, there is a benign microfilarial organism called *Dipetelonemia* that must be distinguished from the heartworm microfilaria *Difilaria*. Care has to be taken to avoid misidentification.

When monthly heartworm prevention came along, confusion set in. This is because the monthly heartworm preventatives themselves are microfilaricidal—that is, they are sometimes used to kill microfilaria. Suddenly it was possible to have more occult infections than before, and **antigen** testing was developed as a result. In an antigen test, instead of examining the blood for microfilaria, the blood sample is mixed with a chemical reagent that binds to any antigen present. A color change on the snap test indicates a positive result. This type of testing quickly became popular. It is highly accurate (missing only those cases where fewer than three heartworms are present in the dog), simple to perform without all the lengthy preparation of the previous test method, and best of all, requires only a few drops of blood. Once this type of test became available, it soon became the test of choice for most veterinarians, especially as monthly heartworm preventative became the most popular choice of prevention as well.

The monthly heartworm preventatives come in several forms. There are the familiar chewy treats given as a pill once a month, as well a whole host of topical agents that are absorbed through the skin. Monthly and topical preventatives are designed to eliminate the L3 larvae in the first 45 days after exposure. If given every thirty days on schedule, the life cycle of the heartworm is effectively halted. Once the L3 larvae change into the L4 stage, the monthly preventative may not be effective in interrupting the life cycle. The L4 form is then free to go on and develop into adult heartworms.

Concerns Over Giving Preventatives

What are some of the concerns that people have with giving heartworm preventative?

Many pet owners state that they do not live in an area of high mosquito activity. This argument is like saying that your child does not need to wear a bicycle safety helmet because there are seldom any cars on your road. All it takes is one mosquito carrying the infective L3 larva to spread the disease. Even if your immediate area has a low local incidence, you can't discount the fact that many people travel with their dogs. Demographic studies show the spread of heartworm disease along the major north-south interstates as dog owners travel from Canada to Florida every winter and spring. These pets can return to your hometown carrying heartworm disease with them.

Owners of small indoor housedogs mistakenly assume that their pets are not outside enough to be at risk. While their chance of exposure may be less than an outdoor dog, small housedogs are at greater risk of developing more serious complications due to the relative size of their hearts.

What about the safety of the medications themselves? The original daily heartworm medications were meant to keep a steady level of preventative in the dog's bloodstream to eliminate microfilaria as they are deposited. If two consecutive days of medication were missed, the microfilaria could penetrate deeper tissues and were no longer responsive to the daily medication. The microfilaria could then continue their merry way to develop into adult heartworms, all the while you thought you were protecting your dog because you remembered and re-started the medication.

In addition, there were sometimes serious side effects with the older products. Many people developed a fear of these products due to a history of adverse reactions. Some of the older, daily preventatives were combination products designed to control hookworm outbreaks, but the added ingredient to prevent hookworms was implicated in causing hepatitis, sterility, and certain blood disorders. None of those daily combination products are on the market anymore.

About thirty years ago, monthly heartworm medications were introduced and have proven to be a safe and effective means of preventing heartworm disease. The original monthly preventative had ivermectin as the active ingredient. The amount of ivermectin in a heartworm tablet is exceedingly small and is considered safe for those breeds with ivermectin sensitivities. In addition to collies, many other breeds of dogs can have ivermectin sensitivity, which leads to the adage, "White Feet, Don't Treat," referring to the fact so many dogs with white socks seem to have this sensitivity.

This doesn't mean you can't use ivermectin-based heartworm products in these breeds, but it does mean you need to be very cautious in using ivermectin off-label in higher doses in these breeds to treat demodectic mange for example. We know now that these ivermectin-sensitive dogs have the MDR1 gene, which makes them sensitive to a whole host of medications, such as chemotherapy medications, common over the counter anti-diarrhea meds such as loperamide, and antifungal treatments. You can now have your dog tested to see if he carries the MDR1 gene.

I once saw a client put her collie in a coma by administering a dose of the cattle dewormer ivermectin on the advice of her neighbor, which is a thousand times stronger than what's used in heartworm prevention. It was three weeks before the dog recovered sufficiently to stand and walk again. Again, this would not have happened with the amount of ivermectin in canine heartworm preventatives, which is a fraction of the dose in the cattle dewormer. This is another reason you should consult with a veterinarian before taking the advice of a neighbor or someone on social media. Many rescue organizations will use diluted cattle dewormer in an effort to save money, and you can find formulas for dosing online as a result. The last time I had a client who dosed their dog using such a recommendation, they administered 37 times the recommended dose. Please consult your veterinarian before choosing to give something to your dog or manage a health condition on your own!

Reproductive studies have shown no adverse effects of ivermectin on male performance, and these preventatives are considered safe to use during pregnancy as well. Many ivermectin-based products have an added ingredient, pyrantel pamoate, to help prevent the spread of hookworms and roundworms. Pyrantel considered a safe dewormer for puppies and kittens, although we are starting to see some parasite resistance to it.

Other monthly tablets may contain milbemycin oxime as their active ingredient. Milbemycin is effective in controlling or eliminating several other internal parasites with no added dewormer. Milbemycin is the only monthly product that will help control whipworms. For some people living in the south where intestinal parasites are deadly to kenneled dogs, it is the best means of controlling a wide variety of parasites. Milbemycin appears to have very few side effects, although there are some anecdotal reports of epileptic dogs being more likely to seizure on the same day that *any* monthly heartworm prevention is given. If you have a dog that seizures, you may want to discuss with your veterinarian the use of other available products.

There are some heartworm preventatives that are topical agents and must be absorbed through the skin to be effective. Some of these products also function as flea control, but truthfully, ticks are such an issue in our area, that I recommend clients use products that will prevent all three parasites instead. The ability to effectively apply the medication (as well as the presence of small children in the home) may cause some people to choose the monthly pill method instead. Coming from an area where so many dogs have heartworms, I prefer an oral product over a topical one, so I can be sure the correct amount of medication gets into the dog.

Another recent development in heartworm prevention is the advent of an injection given once every twelve months. It must be administered by a veterinarian. Some veterinarians believe that the advantages of continual coverage, during which time no L3 larvae can undergo further development, may be crucial to preventing any tissue damage at all. Others have raised concerns about a product that, once administered, cannot be eliminated or discontinued should adverse reactions occur.

When deciding about the use of heartworm preventatives, there are many to choose from. Be sure to get your veterinarian's input as the importance and efficacy of coverage keeps changing.

There are some concerns that we're starting to see resistance to heartworm preventatives, and as such, newer products are being developed all the time. Some of the more recent products combine flea and tick agents with the heartworm prevention. Some only include a flea agent, which means you still have to use something for tick control, which invariably gets fleas as well. Choosing the right product can be challenging, and it is something you should discuss with your veterinarian.

If you decide not to administer a heartworm preventative product at all, you should have your dog tested every six months. This will allow an infection to be identified at the earliest possible time so treatment can be initiated if needed. Dogs that test with a weak positive result on an antigen test **and who are also microfilaria negative** can be safely placed on some forms of the monthly heartworm preventative and may be candidates for what is known as the slow kill method. This method of treatment is not recommended by the American Heartworm Association, but it may be necessary to consider in some patients for health or economic reasons. Some of these dogs may revert to a negative status and do not require the arsenic-based treatments. The same can be done for a microfilaria negative dog that is too ill or old to undergo heartworm treatment. Putting the dog on a heartworm preventative will keep the dog from developing additional worms and eliminate the source of microfilaria so that the dog will not be a risk to other dogs in the area, but it will not treat the adult worms in the heart.

Because giving a heartworm positive dog heartworm medication can trigger a life-threatening anaphylactic if microfilaria are present, such actions must only be taken with veterinary supervision.

What About Cats?

Do cats get heartworms? Yes, they do, but since they are not the natural host, they are not as susceptible to heartworms as dogs are. Also, sometimes they have fewer than three adult female worms in the heart, which means they might not test positive on a heartworm antigen test. Currently, there is no specific treatment for heartworm disease in cats other than managing their severe symptoms.

Cats have **pulmonary inflammatory macrophages** in their lungs, which causes them to react strongly to the presence of heartworms in their bodies. As a species, cats are prone to asthma, but when they have heartworms, they frequently have pronounced symptoms of asthma that don't always respond to treatment as expected. Unlike dogs, vomiting is often a sign of heartworm disease in cats.

The incidence of heartworms in cats is much lower than that of dogs, however. Because there are no effective treatment options and heartworm disease in cats is frequently fatal, many vets recommend year-round heartworm prevention in cats. If you live in an area where heartworms are a major problem for dogs, then your cat is at risk too, and you should consider preventatives.

Treatment Of an Active Infection

Treatment of an active heartworm infection is a multi-stage process. In the past, treatment plans were designed to kill the adult heartworms first and then follow up with a second treatment to destroy the microfilaria. The protocols have changed with the advent of newer medications. These days, once a dog has been diagnosed and the appropriate testing has been done to determine if the infected dog is healthy enough to undergo treatment, most patients are started on the antibiotic doxycycline prior to the first heartworm treatment injection. The doxycycline is used to kill a bacterial organism that lives inside the heartworms, thus making the worms more susceptible to the drug treatment when it is given.

The dogs are also started on an ivermectin-based heartworm preventative to kill off the microfilaria. This needs to be done in a hospital setting with strict supervision, as it is not uncommon for anaphylactic shock to occur about six to eight hours post administration of a heartworm pill to a positive dog due to the massive die-off of microfilaria. If the dog doesn't have any adverse reactions, it will remain on heartworm preventative once a month during the rest of the treatment. After an appropriate period, the dog will be hospitalized and given a series of arsenic-based injections to kill the adult heartworms, usually four weeks apart.

Although the newer treatments are associated with fewer serious side effects than what was available just ten years ago, the treatment and recovery phase are fraught with potential complications. The products used to kill the adult heartworms are still arsenic-based compounds. During the four-week interval between treatment for the adult heartworms and clearing the microfilaria, the dogs must be kept strictly confined. Treatment of the adult heartworms does not result in their immediate elimination from the body. The adult worms die and are slowly broken down and removed by the tissues of the body (**resorbed**). Excessive excitement or activity during this recovery period can cause a mass of dead or dying worms to shift suddenly out of the heart and into the lungs, resulting in respiratory distress and death.

The possibility of anaphylactic shock is why you should **never** administer any heartworm preventative to a dog that has not been properly tested and known to be free of heartworm disease unless under veterinary supervision.

Some people advocate the so-called "slow-kill" method of treating heartworms, which involves putting the dogs on doxycycline and heartworm preventative without giving the arsenic injections and seeing if, over time, the dogs cease to test positive. The American Heartworm Association doesn't think this is an appropriate treatment, as it does nothing to treat the adult worms in the dog and the damage caused by these worms continues to be a factor. There may be several reasons why your vet might suggest the slow kill option over the traditional treatment. The cost and the health of the patient are just two factors to consider.

In Conclusion...

Heartworm disease is a devastating condition with severe physical complications. It will rob your dog of his vitality and shorten his life. While the medications to treat an active heartworm infection are much less toxic than they used to be, they are still strong chemicals with the potential for serious reactions. The potential side effects of these treatments are rare compared to the devastation that is caused by heartworms themselves. More importantly, preventative medication is something that you can do for your pet that is easy, safe, and in some cases helps control other serious parasite problems as well.

Discuss with your veterinarian which heartworm preventative is most appropriate for you and your pet. Be your pet's advocate as well as an educated consumer. Keeping an open mind and a balanced, responsible, educated approach to veterinary care will only benefit the dogs we love. Heartworm disease is extremely preventable. Of all the decisions we make on behalf of our pets, choosing to use some small preventative measures can save you a ton of heartache in the end.

For more information contact: www.heartwormsociety.org

Section 8: Lyme Disease in Dogs

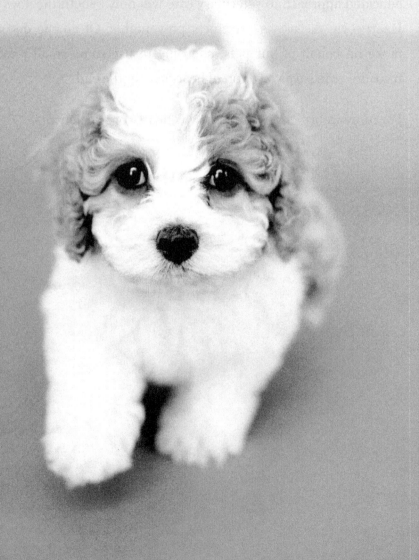

Lyme Disease in Dogs

Lyme disease is something that most people in the U.S. are familiar with these days, thanks to the growing number of cases being identified and reported since the 1980s. It is now considered to be the most common arthropod-borne disease in the country in humans. (Arthropods are organisms like insects, spiders, and ticks with a jointed body and chitinous outer coating.) It is rapidly becoming one of the most common arthropod-borne diseases in dogs as well.

What Causes Lyme Disease?

The causative agent, *Borrelia burgdorferi*, is a spirochete, a spiral shaped bacterium that is also related to the organisms leptospirosis and syphilis. Recently, another Borrelia species has been identified that can cause Lyme-like symptoms, *Borrelia mayonii*. These organisms are transmitted primarily through the bite of an infected tick of the Ixodes family. Bear with me here: the way the disease is spread has implications for why it is not easily controlled. The Ixodes ticks have a two-year life cycle that involves various hosts. These hosts that serve as a reservoir for the Borrelia spirochetes and transmit them to the immature and adult ticks for spread to the next host. The adult female tick lays over two thousand eggs in the early spring. These hatch and mature as larvae, feeding on primarily white-footed mice in the Northeastern US. The white-footed mouse is a handsome brown mouse with a white underbelly and paws. This mouse can harbor the spirochetes for an extended period without becoming ill itself.

The larvae molt into nymphs the following spring. The nymphs move onto a wide variety of hosts, including humans and dogs. In the fall of the second year, they mature into adults, and their host of choice becomes the white-tailed deer. Both nymphs and adult Ixodes ticks can spread Borrelia, but it is believed that the adults are the more effective vector and that exposure during the fall and early spring is most likely to result in clinical disease. It is also believed that repeated exposure may be necessary to cause the development of actual disease. As many as 50% of adult Ixodes ticks in the Northeast may be carrying *B. burgdorferi*.

Is Lyme everywhere?

Lyme disease is a regional problem, limited primarily to the Northeast and Mid-Atlantic States. A small percentage of Lyme disease has been reported in the Midwest and California, but while these areas have species of Ixodes ticks, the important host reservoirs are not the same as in the Northeast. In areas where the nymphs feed primarily on lizards verses white-footed mice, the incidence of Lyme disease is exceptionally low (1-4%). Various environmental factors are going to play a role in the local incidence of *B. burgdorferi* as well. If it is a "good" year for the mice and deer (abundant food supply), then the incidence of Lyme disease has the potential to increase. Ixodes ticks are active in weather at 35 degrees F and above. That means for many areas, tick control should be year-round. The nymphs are so small that they can easily be overlooked on either a dog or a human being.

Prevention

The single most important thing that you can do to prevent Lyme disease is to keep your dog as tick-free as humanly possible. New products for tick control are coming out every day, so it's best to discuss with your veterinarian the products recommended for your area and specific needs.

Rapid removal/death of the ticks is also important. In the past, it was believed the ticks needed to be attached for at least 24-48 hours before the spirochetes begin transmission. Newer studies indicate it may take far less time than that, so bottom line, practice good tick control.

Programs to control ticks in the mouse and deer population have met with limited success. Repellents containing DEET or permethrin are available for use in animals but need to be used judiciously because of the potential for toxicity. Pets (as well as their humans) should be checked daily for ticks. Do not assume that your control is 100%. The nymphs are so tiny you might never even see them. Any pet showing clinical signs of fever and joint pain should be evaluated for potential Lyme disease.

Symptoms And Diagnosis

Researchers think that only 5% of exposed dogs go on to develop clinical disease. There are four criteria that must be met to make a diagnosis:

1. There must be a history of exposure (ticks, travel to region).

2. Typical clinical signs of fever, joint pain/enlargement.

3. Positive titer (see Section 12 for more information on titers).

4. Prompt response to antibiotics.

Dogs with Lyme disease typically present with a moderate to marked fever as well as generalized joint pain and lethargy. Quite often, their owners will describe the dog as "walking on eggshells." Enlarged lymph nodes and/or enlarged joints may or may not be seen. In the rare case, there may be uveitis—an inflammation of the chamber of the eye. Dogs with uveitis typically show signs of ocular pain: unwillingness to hold the lids open, sensitivity to bright light, and potentially a hazy appearance of the fluid in the eye itself.

The severe neurologic, kidney, and heart problems described in humans with chronic Lyme disease are not as common in dogs; however, fatal nephritis has been reported, particularly in Labradors. For some reason, when Labs get Lyme, they can get sicker than other breeds.

It is important to note that a positive titer alone does not always determine the presence of disease. A dog may have a positive titer through exposure that did not result in disease. The original vaccine available for use in dogs was a whole cell bacterin—meaning they used the entire organism in the vaccine—this vaccine would also cause a positive titer indistinguishable from active disease or exposure. Vaccinating for Lyme disease in the past has been controversial, as the mechanism of the chronic disease state is not well understood. The risks of the complications of Lyme disease, combined with the safety of the newer recombinant technology vaccines, mean vaccination is usually recommended in areas where Lyme is prevalent.

Unfortunately, sometimes you can miss the acute signs of Lyme disease. Your dog may be ill for only a day or two, and by the time you decide to call your vet, your dog is better again. It's not unusual for these patients to wind up with widespread arthritis or kidney issues later on, so annual screening via the combination heartworm/tick disease snap tests may be useful. If your dog tests positive on a snap test, your vet may recommend a confirmatory titer or suggest treatment, especially if your dog has no previous history of testing positive.

To date, Lyme disease is not typically seen in cats, though they can get other tick-borne diseases. Cytauxzoonosis is a tick disease of bobcats, and it is frequently fatal in pet cats, so tick control is important for your house tiger too.

The disease course differs in dogs versus humans in some key areas:

- The owner of the dog seldom sees a rash.

- Incubation can be as long as 5 months in dogs.

- Most animals will present with fever and joint pain as the primary complaint.

- Serious complications, such as neurologic, cardiac, and kidney involvement, are not seen as frequently in dogs as in humans.

Treatment

The antibiotic of choice for treatment of Lyme is doxycycline or minocycline. Amoxicillin and other drugs in the penicillin class can be used in pregnant bitches or puppies that have immature teeth due to the effects of doxycycline in these situations. Doxycycline is thought to have a direct effect on decreasing the development of the arthritis complex. Because titers do not correlate well with response to treatment, monitoring for a decreasing titer is not as useful in this disease as in some of the other tick-borne diseases (such as Rocky Mountain Spotted Fever). It is not unusual for dogs to have as many as 2-3 recurrent episodes of joint pain and fever from a single "exposure" of Lyme disease because of the long incubation period. The recurrent episodes seem to be as responsive to antibiotics as the first time but may be an indication that a longer course of antibiotics could be beneficial. Dogs that have had their spleens surgically removed for whatever reason may be at higher risk of developing any of the tick-borne diseases, including Ehrlichia, Rocky Mountain Spotted Fever, and tick paralysis, as the spleen is part of the immune system.

In most cases, dogs respond to an appropriate antibiotic within 24 hours. Therapy must usually be continued for 2-4 weeks, but even the length of therapy is controversial. Some clinicians feel that because of the long incubation period in dogs, a longer course of antibiotics may be warranted.

Dogs with uveitis or other immune mediated inflammatory conditions may benefit from treatment with corticosteroids in conjunction with an appropriate antibiotic, but the need for steroids will vary with the individual and may mask signs or prolong the incubation period.

It is not believed that pregnant bitches can transmit the disease to unborn puppies; however, care must be taken when treating the pregnant bitch with certain antibiotics. Tetracycline and related products, the drugs of choice in treating Lyme disease, should be used with caution in pregnant bitches or in puppies with immature teeth, as it will permanently stain the enamel of the developing adult teeth. That said, stained teeth aren't lethal. Sometimes you must use what drugs are available.

Conclusion

Lyme disease in dogs carries a favorable prognosis for complete recovery. Because it can present with so many different clinical signs, you aren't going to find it if you aren't looking for it. Whether or not to vaccinate for Lyme depends on the prevalence of the disease in your area. Prevalence can change, too. Due to the changing climate, we're seeing new species and diseases move into our area we've never had to deal with before. Talk with your veterinarian before deciding whether to vaccinate. Most vaccine protocols recommend starting the Lyme series at 9 weeks of age along with the distemper/parvo vaccine and then annually thereafter.

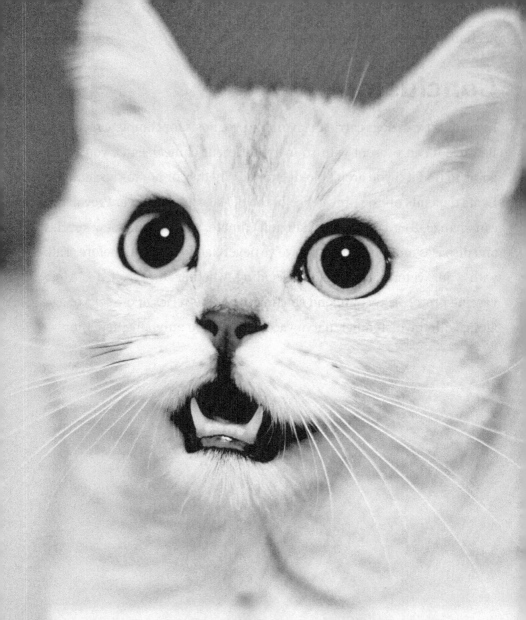

Section 9: Tests of
the Eyes

Tests Of the Eyes

No, your veterinarian is not going to hold up an eye chart and ask your dog to read the top line! But there are some basic eye tests that you should be familiar with in the exam room. Your vet may not run most of them as part of the minimum database, but there will be situations in which performing these tests might be part of your pet's examination.

There are two things to remember about the eyes:

- First, there are so many distinct parts to the eye that it has its own vocabulary and terms specific to discussing ocular conditions. I'll try not to overwhelm with too much terminology!

- Second, like joints, eyes are mostly a closed, protected system. This means while it is difficult for infections to get started within the eye, it is equally difficult for medications to penetrate the eye as well. That can make certain types of conditions challenging to medicate and correct.

Eye Examination

Initially, your vet is going to examine the external structures of the eye, looking at the clarity and appearance of the corneal surface, as well as examining the surrounding conjunctival tissues. A red, inflamed-looking eye is going to send up a red flag for your vet, who might need to do further testing.

With the use of an ophthalmoscope, your vet will be able to examine the internal structures of the eye, looking for signs of cataracts, assessing the health of the retinas and the optic disk, as well as looking for signs of **uveitis**, which is inflammation of several different pigmented components inside the eye, including the iris. The iris is the part of the eye that grants eye color. A change in the color of the iris can indicate the presence of uveitis.

Damage to the cornea

If your vet suspects that the cornea, the external surface of the eye, is scratched or damaged in some way, she might perform a **fluorescein dye test.** In this test, your vet will place a small amount of dye on the cornea and then wash the dye out again. The dye will stick to any part of the cornea that is damaged. Because the dye is fluorescent under a blacklight, this piece of equipment may be used to look for subtle dye retention. A corneal ulcer is usually deeper than a scratch and may potentially penetrate all the way into the chamber of the eye. Determining the presence or absence of corneal damage is crucial before deciding on certain types of eye medication. **Medications containing steroids should never be used in an eye with a corneal ulcer.**

You should never use leftover medication from one pet to another without consulting with your veterinarian. When I was a student in vet school, I was assigned a horse who had been blinded by his owner's decision to use her dog's eye ointment on her horse instead of contacting a vet. The steroid-based eye ointment caused the eye, which had been scratched, to develop a "melting" corneal ulcer. In this condition, the damaged cornea begins to disintegrate under the influence of the steroid and can eventually end in the rupture of the globe itself.

This is not to say that there is there is never an appropriate use for a steroid-based medication. One of my German Shepherds had to take steroid eye drops to control an immune-mediated deposition of pigment on the cornea called **pannus**, but the need for steroids must be determined by veterinary examination. A corneal ulcer should always be ruled out before using steroids in the eye.

Dry Eye

If your dog presents to the veterinarian with exceptionally "goopy" eyes, having a thick green discharge in the absence of an eye infection and with leathery looking corneas, your vet may want to run a **Schirmer Tear Test (STT).**

"Dry eye" (canine *keratitis sicca or* KCS) is common in many breeds of dogs (including spaniels and bulldogs) and can also result from hypothyroidism and certain medications. In KCS, the normal tear mechanism is faulty. Tears are made up of a fluid and mucus component. In KCS, the fluid component begins to decrease, resulting in the drying out of the corneal surface.

In the initial stages, this can be hard to notice in dogs that have very dark irises because the corneal surface is not easy to distinguish from the background of the eye. As tear production fails, the mucus component of the tear mechanism begins to over-produce in compensation. The dogs have a constant slimy green covering to their eyes, which re-appears when wiped away. A STT strip is a small piece of filter paper that has been impregnated with a dye and is delineated with markings. This filter paper is placed in the corner of the eye and held in place for sixty seconds. As the tears present in the conjunctiva wick out along the filter paper, it carries the dye out along with it. At the end of sixty seconds, the distance the tears have traveled will indicate whether the tear production is normal or not. Abnormal tear production levels can sometimes be improved with medication when detected early in the disease process. Without treatment, the cornea will become more damaged. It defends itself by becoming leathery and heavily pigmented, resulting in permanent vision loss.

Glaucoma

This is a condition when the **internal pressure of the eye begins to rise**. The eye normally produces a certain amount of thick fluid called the **vitreous humor**. It's called this because when the Greeks first began studying the human body, the different fluids in the body were referred to as "humors," which has nothing to do with being funny! This fluid re-circulates and drains out of the eye through tiny ports called drainage angles. For many reasons, these little ports can become blocked. The eye will continue to produce the vitreous humor, but it will have no way to leave, thus resulting in increasing pressure.

There are many breeds predisposed to glaucoma, and it can also result from trauma, infection, and cancer, or from **lens luxation.** A damaged lens, or one developing cataracts, can sometimes lose its "mooring;" it can become unseated from the supports that keep it suspended in front of the iris. If the lens capsule tears or leaks, then the eye will react to the proteins within the lens capsule as foreign material and cause an intense reaction, the fallout of which can block the drainage angles. Sometimes no obvious cause for the glaucoma can be identified.

Breeds at risk for developing glaucoma:

- Cocker Spaniels

- Most terriers, but especially the Jack Russell

- Many of the Northern breeds, such as Siberian Huskies

- Poodles

- Beagles

- Chows

- Basset hounds

- Dalmatians

- Corgis

- Westies

- Border Collies

- Labradors

This list is by no means complete. Bottom line, glaucoma has been diagnosed in every breed.

Cats, while less likely to get glaucoma, can also develop it, and Persians and Siamese cats are more prone than other species.

Any red eye should be checked for glaucoma. Animals that typically develop glaucoma may show evidence of pain around the face and eyes and redness of the eyeball and surrounding tissues. In late stages, the eye can enlarge dramatically due to buildup of the internal pressure. If the pressure is severe, permanent damage to the retina occurs, even if you can get the pressure down again with medication. If you have a lens luxation, the loose lens may need to be surgically removed. Sometimes enucleation (removal of the eye) is the only way to manage the pressure and pain. It is far better to screen for glaucoma and start treatment early than to attempt to rescue the eye on an emergency basis.

Uveitis

As we mentioned earlier, **uveitis** is an inflammation of the uvea: the pigmented part of the eye, which includes the iris, the ciliary body, and choroid, which is where all the blood vessels are. In cases of uveitis, the

internal pressure of the eye can fall. Decreased ocular pressure in an inflamed eye is often a good indicator of uveitis. Many times, after the initial drop in pressures due to infection, blockage of drainage angles due to inflammatory cells and debris can result in secondary glaucoma. In addition to a change in color of the iris, the inflammatory cells are sometimes visible when you shine a light sideways through the front of the eye. Picture dust motes in a beam of sunlight. That's how uveitis can appear. The whole visible chamber of the eye can look cloudy in the right light.

Checking eye pressures is a standard part of every eye exam and you might want to request it as part of an annual exam if you have one of the high-risk breeds or a history of glaucoma in your dog's bloodlines. It is also recommended as part of a senior/geriatric exam and in cases of head trauma.

NEWSFLASH

A "red" eye should always be treated as an emergency and be examined as soon as possible!

Section 10: Thyroid Testing

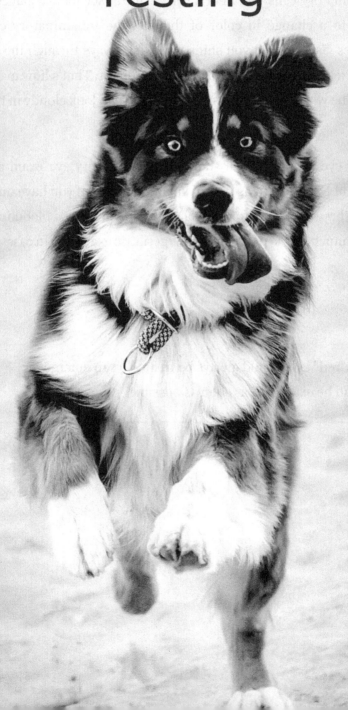

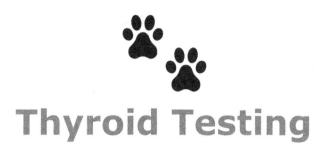

Thyroid Testing

The thyroid is a busy little gland. It secretes thyroid hormone in sufficient quantities to run a wide variety of systems. The normal functioning thyroid gland is responsible for a stable metabolism, normal skin and cell turnover, and a healthy immune system.

The main hormones produced by the thyroid gland are thyroxine or tetraiodothyronine (T4) and triiodothyronine (T3). A thyroid function test assesses the level of these two hormones. A third hormone, the Thyroid Stimulating Hormone (TSH) is produced by the pituitary gland, and basically regulates the thyroid. A full thyroid "panel" tests for this hormone, too.

Testing Thyroid Levels

Many in-house lab machines can test thyroid levels now, but they usually only test for T4 levels, as opposed to the complete array of hormones created by the thyroid gland. While testing for T4 levels is accurate most of the time, 25% of the time, T4 levels will be normal even when the patient is **hypothyroid**, the condition when there is not enough circulating or available thyroid hormone in the body. It can be challenging to determine whether a dog needs thyroid supplementation or not, and excess thyroid hormone creates another set of complications and issues to deal with.

Certain medications, most notably steroids, anticonvulsant therapy, and certain antibiotics can affect thyroid levels. While they act by different mechanisms, the general effect is to decrease thyroid hormone levels or the body's effective use of thyroid hormones. When possible, if I suspect a thyroid problem, I try to draw my blood sample before initiating such medications, or else I wait until at least two weeks after the discontinuation of these medications to prevent skewing the test results.

Chronic disease and other non-thyroidal illnesses can result in lowered thyroid levels as well (also known as **sick euthyroid syndrome**). A dog may sometimes be clinically hypothyroid in appearance but have normal thyroid levels because of an inability to access the thyroid hormones and metabolize them properly. Your veterinarian might suggest a trial on thyroid supplement despite normal or borderline thyroid values. If there is a response to supplementation, a repeat of the thyroid profile should be performed (four to six hours after the morning pill). If it is decided to discontinue supplementation because the response is uncertain, then you should wait four to six weeks before checking the levels again to avoid a falsely depressed measurement. While a dog is receiving supplementation, the thyroid gland will naturally produce less of its own hormone amounts. You need to wait at least this long to allow the gland to restart normal production, if indeed it can do so. To confuse the issue further, sighthounds and giant breed dogs typically have lower than average thyroid levels. You must be careful in interpreting thyroid values in these. These dogs, such as Salukis, Whippets, and Greyhounds, may have lower resting thyroid levels and still be perfectly normal.

I am not going to discuss in detail the interpretation of thyroid test results because even a trained endocrinologist, when confronted with certain test results and clinical signs, will often suggest a trial on medication. What you need to know is this: it may be necessary to send your dog's blood sample for an appropriate **thyroid panel** rather than just testing for T4 levels if you are trying to diagnose thyroid disease for the first time in a dog. Usually this means sending the sample sent out to an outside laboratory rather than being performed in-house on a chemistry machine. A full thyroid profile typically examines total T4 and T3 levels, free T4 and T3 levels, T3 and T4 autoantibodies, and thyroid stimulating hormone (TSH) levels.

This is because dogs can be hypothyroid with normal total T4 levels, and T4 values are the most likely to be suppressed by sick euthyroid syndrome. Free T4 levels (FT4) represent the biologically available hormone and are therefore more reflective of the true condition. FT4 is less affected by sick euthyroid syndrome. The body converts T4 to T3, so it is useful to see these levels as well. Since most hypothyroid cases are caused by an autoimmune thyroiditis, having the autoantibody levels is a significant piece of information to have during initial screening tests.

TSH levels frequent rise in cases of thyroid deficiency, as the body is trying to compensate for the lack of hormone by triggering the gland to make more. Once a dog has been supplemented over time, these levels should return to a more normal state as supplementation is thought to interrupt the feedback loop between thyroid stimulating hormone and the autoantibody formation.

T4 levels alone are perfectly fine for monitoring therapy or diagnosing **hyperthyroidism** in cats. Many clinics can perform in-house T4 levels, and so this is often their first (and less expensive) choice for diagnostics, but if there is any question in your mind about the results, then a full panel is indicated.

Thyroid stimulating hormone (TSH) is released by the pituitary gland and stimulates the release of thyroid hormones by that gland. If you have a dog with normal or borderline thyroid levels but the TSH is elevated, then the body is working extremely hard to maintain those levels. A high TSH level will always makes me look more closely at the rest of the panel results. I also pay special attention to the possibility of other endocrine or autoimmune problems when I identify a case of hypothyroidism.

The Underactive Thyroid: Hypothyroidism

Let's consider the following cases:

Case # 1:

"Buffy" is a 7-year-old female spayed cocker spaniel that weighs seventy-five pounds, with twenty-five pounds being a more appropriate weight. She looks like an ottoman: a short, squat dog shaped like a rectangle with a leg at each corner. She shuffles into the room. Buffy's owner is seeking a second opinion on chronic skin and ear infections. The dog's skin is greasy and smelly, while her coat is sparse and nearly non-existent along her back and sides. The hair is brittle and pulls out easily without any effort. Buffy's facial skin folds hang like that of a Basset hound. Her whole expression is one of great tragedy—a canine Eeyore. No one can understand why she is so overweight since she hardly eats anything. She is extremely sensitive to the cold; she is described as sleeping on the heat vents and so close to the wood stove it is a wonder she hasn't been burned.

Case # 2:

"Rusty" is a 7-year-old male neutered Doberman. He is plump but in good overall health with a dull but otherwise normal coat. Rusty has a rear leg lameness that cannot be isolated to a particular joint. His regular veterinarian suspected a cruciate injury but was not able to confirm this, nor does Rusty seem to respond to pain medication and rest. Referral to specialist garnered a presumptive diagnosis of Wobblers syndrome (an instability of the cervical vertebrae resulting in impingement on the nerves in the spinal cord) and a recommendation for an expensive corrective procedure. A third opinion at the vet school did not support the diagnosis of Wobblers, and the surgery was not recommended.

Case # 3:

"Casey" is a 5-year-old intact male cocker spaniel. He is of normal weight and his coat is in excellent condition. Casey began to have difficulty picking up and chewing his food over the course of the last week and has rapidly gotten worse. At time of presentation, Casey is unable to close his mouth properly and his tongue is hanging out of his mouth. Over the next two days, Casey loses the ability to drink or eat anything at all. Lab work does not indicate any sign of infection.

Analysis

Now, what if I asked you to pick out the hypothyroid dog from among these cases? Well, case number one should send up warning bells for most of us—this is the classic (if exaggeratedly so) presentation for canine hypothyroidism. This condition is typically seen in middle-aged to older dogs, there are breed predispositions, and it is more often seen in females than males. But what if I told you that all three cases were examples of hypothyroidism—and that hypothyroidism was the underlying cause of their primary complaint?

Buffy's thyroid levels were almost non-existent. Supplementation was crucial to solving her underlying skin problems. Rusty ended up being tested for hypothyroidism almost a year after the "lameness" began. The lameness resolved after initiation of supplementation. In the most rewarding case, Casey was rapidly deteriorating while the thyroid test results were still pending. His owners tearfully requested that we euthanize him. Having nothing to lose on a long shot, we persuaded them to delay the decision temporarily while we started Casey on supplementation until the test results came back. Miraculously, within forty-eight hours of starting the thyroid supplement, Casey was able to swallow and partially close his mouth. After a week, he was able to move his mouth normally again. All three dogs had abnormal thyroid levels on testing, but more importantly, they also responded to thyroid supplementation.

Too little thyroid hormone — hypothyroidism — can result in abnormal weight gain, a dull, brittle or vanishing hair coat, abnormally thickened and /or pigmented skin, and dull mentality, fearful behavior and/or aggression, as well as seizures.

Dogs that are hypothyroid often have repeated infections (especially skin infections) due to a weakened immune system and can develop abnormal tear production leading to a condition called dry eye or **keratoconjunctivitis sicca** (KCS). They can also develop lipid (fatty) deposits on the surface of the corneas and develop uveitis or secondary glaucoma because of fat deposits in the eye. They are often extremely sensitive to the cold and seek warm environments. Intact (unspayed) females will often not cycle normally or have fertility issues and poor survival of pups in a litter. The heart rate of these dogs is often abnormally slow and there can be thinning of the heart muscle as well.

Hypothyroid dogs can also develop **peripheral neuropathies**. A peripheral neuropathy is a disorder of a nerve that is not part of the central nervous system like the spinal cord. Instead, it can affect nerves in the limbs, as in Rusty's mystery "lameness" or facial nerves as in

Casey's strange paralysis. Facial nerve paralysis, also known as Bell's palsy, is rarely seen in hypothyroid dogs, but I used these examples here to show you how a dog may not have all the classic signs of hypothyroidism and still warrant testing.

Hypothyroidism is the most common endocrine disorder in dogs. Primary hypothyroidism usually occurs because of an immune-mediated thyroiditis (which may be heritable) or because of idiopathic atrophy of the gland. In immune-meditated thyroiditis, the thyroid gland is infiltrated by lymphocytes and plasma cells (much the same as immune-mediated inflammatory bowel disease). This slowly obliterates the normal thyroid gland and replaces it with fibrous tissue. In idiopathic atrophy, the gland withers away and is replaced by fatty tissue.

In rare cases, hypothyroidism is secondary to cancer infiltrating the gland itself, or involving the pituitary gland, which (among other things) controls the release of thyroid stimulating hormone (TSH).

Because of the potentially inherited nature of this condition, affected animals should not be used for breeding. The list of most affected breeds is quite long and varies depending on your source. In my experience, the most common breeds affected are American Cocker Spaniels, Chows, Shetland Sheepdogs, Dobermans, Miniature Schnauzers, Dachshunds, and Golden Retrievers, but in general, it tends to affect mid-to-large breed dogs more commonly than toy breeds and is more common in middle-aged female dogs rather than young, male dogs.

Hypothyroidism: Treatment

Once diagnosed, the treatment is supplementation in the form of a pill that is usually given twice daily. Older dogs and sighthounds are usually started off at the lower end of the dose range. After three months, I will test again and adjust this dosage if needed. If the supplementation results in normal thyroid levels, but the patient still has clinical signs, then that's my cue to consider other causes of the symptoms instead of assuming they are all thyroid related.

The Overactive Thyroid: Hyperthyroidism

Abnormally elevated levels of thyroid hormone can be very detrimental as well. **Hyperthyroidism** is rarely seen naturally in the dog but commonly occurs in cats. In dogs, the most probable cause of hyperthyroidism is excessive supplementation. Supplementation needs can change with age and physical condition, which is why is it necessary to periodically check thyroid levels on dogs that have been determined to be hypothyroid. Or if your dog was sick euthyroid, once the underlying problem was resolved, then thyroid supplementation was no longer necessary.

Excessive thyroid levels can cause extreme weight loss in the face of an almost frantic appetite. Animals can experience **cachexia**, which is a state of catabolic energy drain where the body is burning itself up due to an excessive need for fuel. Cachexia is not limited to hyperthyroidism, however. Cancer, heart disease, and starvation can all cause the same physical signs. Excessive thyroid levels result in hypertension as well as heart damage due to the excessive metabolic rate these animals experience. Animals with hyperthyroidism have high blood pressure and can experience sudden retinal detachment as a result.

Hyperthyroidism is a common condition in geriatric cats because of a tumor of the thyroid gland. In 80-90% of cases, it is a benign tumor that is secreting thyroid hormone in excessive amounts, but on rare occasions, it can be a malignant carcinoma. Sometimes, the tumor is not directly associated with the gland itself, but it has originated somewhere else in the body, where it may or may not be readily identified.

The excessive thyroid hormone production has toxic effects on the metabolism. Most hyperthyroid cats have an elevated heart rate and blood pressure. Many have heart murmurs as well. Most are dropping weight rapidly, despite having a good appetite: in fact, many clients delay bringing their cats in because the cats are eating so well that they assume nothing can be wrong. About ten percent of the time, however, hyperthyroid cats will *lose* their appetite. In the late stages of the disease, these cats can be extremely thin and have concurrent cardiomyopathy. Many clients report unusual activity and increased vocalization. One of my friends told me her aged cat attacked a stuffed doll that had been on her bed for years and tore its face off! I recommended she have her cat checked for hyperthyroidism, and lo and behold, that was his problem.

Some hyperthyroid cats may have chronic vomiting or diarrhea for several years before hyperthyroidism is diagnosed. Many will have nails that grow abnormally thick and fast, sometimes growing around into the footpads.

The Link to Feeding Fish to Cats

The incidence of hyperthyroidism in cats is growing and has been associated with PBDEs, which are fire retardant chemicals that can be found in high concentrations in some fish (also in furniture coverings and house dust). Fish-based food allergies are also quite common in cats.

It's likely because the big, deep-water, wild-caught fish are at the top of the food chain, and thus concentrate toxins and heavy metals (including mercury) as well as PCBs, pesticides, and other toxins. Ocean whitefish, mackerel, shark, and swordfish are among the most heavily contaminated. The FDA advises women of child-bearing age and children to avoid them entirely and recommends only one serving of albacore tuna per week due to its high mercury levels. Human-grade tuna is severely deficient in Vitamin A and should never be used as a food substitute for cats, although it can be used as an occasional treat or if you are trying to tempt the appetite of a sick cat. If these fish are dangerous to *children*, then cats, by virtue of being smaller, are at even higher risk for toxicity.

Due to climate change, a neurotoxin produced by algae called *domoic acid* is increasing in concentration in fish, clams, and mussels caught in coastal waters. The American Society of Nephrology reports that domoic acid damages kidneys at a much lower level than is needed to cause brain damage. Given that fish is used in a filler in almost all cat food, is it any wonder that the incidence of kidney disease and hyperthyroidism in cats is on the rise? I try to look for foods that do not include fish in the first five ingredients, but it isn't easy to find. Before you decide to cook for your cat, be advised that cats have extremely specific amino acid requirements from their diet (which is why you frequently see mention of taurine or carnitine supplementation on the labels). If you get it wrong, you can cause serious metabolic harm to your cat, including the development of dilated cardiomyopathy and permanent retinal damage (Science Daily, 2014).

The short version here is try not to feed your cat any fish-based diets.

Treatment

Of all the geriatric cat diseases, hyperthyroidism is the most treatable, provided your cat doesn't also have diabetes or kidney failure. It can still be manageable under those conditions but trickier.

There are three main methods of treatment, all of which are aimed at normalizing the thyroid levels:

- Radioactive iodine therapy

- Surgical removal of the thyroid tumor

- Suppressing the thyroid function with medication

Radioactive Iodine

The gold standard is **radioactive iodine therapy**. With this treatment option, your cat is injected with radioactive iodine, which is selectively taken up by thyroid tissue anywhere in the body, even if your cat has abnormal or ectopic thyroid tissue that is not directly associated with the thyroid gland. The iodine will destroy the thyroid tissue. In some cases, your cat may end up hypothyroid as a result and need supplementation. Radioactive iodine therapy is a referral procedure, and your cat will temporarily be radioactive for a week or so post treatment (not to worry, he won't develop superpowers!), and must remain at the facility with special handling. As such, careful screening must be done prior to treatment to make sure your cat is a suitable candidate for therapy. Once performed, RIT cannot be reversed!

In some cases, a cat's kidney function can become reliant on the elevated blood pressure that results from hyperthyroidism and reversing the thyroid disease can worsen pre-existing kidney disease or make hidden disease symptomatic. This is why most RIT facilities want the cats to have been treated with the oral medications for at least 30 days prior to initiation of radiation therapy to make sure that treatment won't make things worse for the cat. However, all meds must be stopped for a few weeks before RIT begins to ensure the best uptake of the iodine, so the timing must be coordinated between you, your regular vet, and the RIT facility. Unfortunately, the cost and the need to go to a special facility often precludes this form of treatment for many cat owners.

Surgery

Some facilities still offer **surgical removal of the thyroid tumor**. Again, careful pre-surgical screening is needed to calculate the risks of surgery on a geriatric pet, but as far as the surgery itself goes, the thyroid glands are superficial, and the surgery is not an invasive procedure. The surgery has a high success rate unless there is ectopic tissue as well. Ectopic thyroid tissue (hormone producing tissue outside of the usual thyroid gland) can be hard to identify or be located in an inaccessible area, such as the chest. Surgery works best when the thyroid disease is discovered early, and the cat is still in good physical condition. Even though typically only one of the paired thyroid glands is involved, it is recommended that both be removed, as it is not unheard of for the other side to develop problems over time. One of my own cats had thyroid surgery at 16 years of age, but the tumor returned in the other gland when he was 18 and no longer a candidate for surgery.

The biggest complication associated with surgery occurs when the parathyroid glands are disturbed during the procedure. These tiny glands sit on top of the thyroid glands, and care must be taken not to damage or remove them when removing the abnormal thyroid tissue. If the parathyroid glands are damaged, then the cat may develop life-threatening calcium imbalances and need supplementation on an emergency basis. Even though the calcium balance issues are usually self-limiting once the parathyroid glands stabilize, some surgeons prefer only to remove one thyroid gland at a time for this reason. That way, if there are any problems with the parathyroid hormone regulation, then the other parathyroid gland can pick up the slack.

Medication

The third, and most common, method of treating hyperthyroidism is **suppressing the thyroid function with medication**. Methimazole will suppress the thyroid hormone output, and over a period of weeks, the cat's heart rate and blood pressure will return to normal. The cats will start to regain their lost weight, and in many cases, the previous heart disease will be reversible as well. Sometimes, with cats of advanced age or other health problems, methimazole may be the only treatment warranted. Not all cats can tolerate it, however. It can cause vomiting and dermatitis in some cats and can sometimes severely suppress the bone marrow production of new red and white cells.

I recently saw a cat that had been to a referral institution because it had been attacked by a dog. The cat had recovered from the attack but was now severely anemic. The referral institution was adamant about increasing the cat's methimazole, as they felt the thyroid disease wasn't under control. When I assessed the cat, who was so anemic it was in danger of entering into kidney failure, I took it off methimazole altogether until the red cell count improved. Once the anemia stabilized, we gradually re-introduced the medication, with the understanding that we might not be able to treat the cat at full strength. Sometimes, you must settle for less than perfect control due to the potential side effects. It's the equivalent of wetting the trees in the forest rather than completely putting out the fire. The fire is still there but burning at a slower rate.

One of the good things about methimazole therapy, however, is that you can stop it if you run into problems. I put cats on methimazole for several weeks before considering alternative therapies. In part, because it helps bring down the heart rate and blood pressure before potentially undergoing anesthesia, but also because if correcting the thyroid is going to worsen kidney or liver function, I want to know before I set the cat up for an irreversible procedure.

One of the disadvantages of methimazole (aside from having to medicate your cat daily) is that most cats become refractory (resistant) to it over time. So, while it might be an excellent first choice option for a 16-year-old cat, it may not be a good one for a 13-year-old cat. You run the risk of "running out of medication" when you choose that route for managing a younger cat with thyroid disease, forcing you to switch to alternative therapies several years into treatment—with an even older cat—when going with one of the permanent treatments in the first place might have been the better choice.

Having to medicate your cat every day can be difficult. There are various tricks and aids to help you, but if you can't medicate your cat easily, methimazole can be compounded into a topical gel that is applied to the inside of your cat's ear. Ask your vet about it if you don't think you can pill your cat otherwise.

Section 11: ACTH Stim Testing

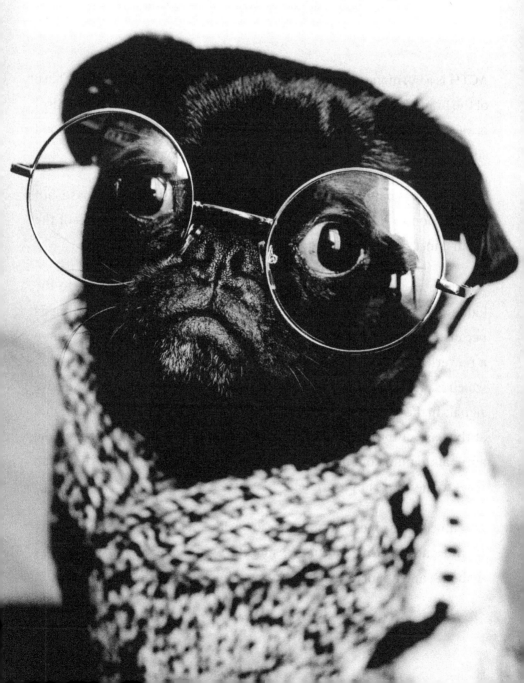

ACTH Stim Testing

ACTH is a hormone made by the pituitary gland, a small gland at the base of the brain. It controls the production of the hormone **cortisol**. Cortisol is released by the adrenal glands and regulates blood pressure, blood sugar, the immune system, and the response to stress.

Stim testing is not one of the routine tests of the minimum database, but the decision to run this test is frequently triggered by the results of the chem panel.

The adrenal glands are small, peanut-sized glands that sit close to the kidneys. The medical term for kidney is "renal," so these are the adrenals because they are next to the kidneys. Get it? For small glands, they serve a powerful function in the body. They are the prime source of cortisol, which is critical for running certain systems. The adrenal glands receive signals in the form of hormones from the pituitary gland, which is located at the base of the brain. The hormones secreted by the pituitary tell the adrenals to pump out more cortisol in times of stress so that the body can react to the stress appropriately.

Too much cortisol can result in serious side effects, such as an inability to concentrate urine normally, muscle wasting, hair loss, secondary diabetes, and an increased sensitivity to infection, to name a few.

Too little cortisol, however, can be imminently life-threatening, as the tiny amounts of cortisol produced by the adrenal glands are critical to maintaining the balance of electrolytes in your body. Because electrolytes are important in so many functions, having an electrolyte imbalance has the potential to kill you quickly.

Hyperadrenocorticism (Cushing's Disease)

Too much cortisol typically results in a thinning or poor-quality hair coat, especially down the middle of the back, and the muscles of the belly thin as well, so the dogs (and more rarely, cats) frequently take on the appearance of a little pot-bellied pig. These animals also lose the ability to concentrate urine, which means usually they are consuming excessive quantities of water and peeing it out as fast as they take it in. This is what most clients bring the dogs in for: they are drinking unusual amounts of water and peeing in the house. Because **hyperadrenocorticism** (or Cushing's disease) is typically a disease of middle-aged and older dogs, clients will often mistake the signs for aging, when in fact, they are abnormal. Cushing's is a common health problem in older dogs. It can be expensive to treat, especially in larger dogs.

These dogs are usually drinking three to four times as much water as normal and cannot concentrate their urine above the specific gravity of water. When we run basic lab work on them, their alkaline phosphatase (ALP or ALKP) is frequently elevated – see section 3.2 for more on this. In fact, ALP elevations of six to twelve times the normal range are possible. Ruling out Cushing's is important when you see this kind of elevation in a senior dog. Just to complicate matters, though, the ALP can be *normal* in Cushing's dogs. Regardless of ALP levels, the inability to concentrate urine (usually the specific gravity of the urine is around 1.010—close to that of pure water) is one of the main signs of Cushing's.

In Cushing's, the body is producing too much cortisol. This is usually the result of a tumor, either in the adrenal gland itself, or in the pituitary gland. A primary adrenal gland tumor that is producing excessive cortisol can sometimes be surgically removed, although this isn't always feasible in an older dog. Most of the time, however, the tumor is pituitary-based, and we don't even have access to it because the pituitary gland sits under the brain. Instead of producing cortisol directly, the pituitary gland produces excess adrenocorticotropic hormone (ACTH). This hormone, in turn, cranks up the adrenals so they can produce high doses of cortisol.

To confirm suspected Cushing's, your vet may order what's called an ACTH stim test to rule out Cushing's as a cause for the **polydipsia** (drinking too much water) and **polyuria** (you guessed it, peeing too much). There are a number of different agents used to run these stim tests, and the products change over time, but first you establish baseline cortisol levels with an initial blood sample. Then, your vet administers an agent that will stimulate adrenals to release cortisol. Depending on the agent used, your pet will need to have multiple blood samples taken during the day. Timing of this is dependent on the agent used to stimulate the cortisol release. Some of the less expensive tests are useful for screening but not for monitoring therapy, so there may be differences in what test is used for which purpose. The low-dose dexamethasone test is highly accurate for screening but not good for monitoring therapy. The ACTH stim test with cortrosyn, a synthetic hormone, is the gold standard for monitoring therapy, but it's less accurate for determining if Cushing's is present in the first place. Suffice to say, the resting cortisol should be in the normal range, and the stimulated cortisol should not exceed a specific amount. Elevations on the stim test confirm the likelihood of Cushing's.

Hypoadrenocorticism: Addison's Disease

The ACTH stim test is also used, however, to diagnose the reverse of Cushing's, which is called Addison's disease, or **hypoadrenocorticism**. In this case, the body is not producing enough cortisol or the special mineralocorticoids necessary to keep your electrolytes in balance. The hallmark of Addison's is weakness and collapse due to the derangement of the electrolytes, and it's frequently associated with vomiting and diarrhea. Because of this, Addison's is often misdiagnosed at first because when a patient comes in with acute vomiting and diarrhea, they frequently are given fluids, which temporarily re-balances the electrolytes. However, the balance can't be maintained without the trace amounts of cortisol made by the body, so the patient crashes once more.

On the basic lab work, these dogs usually have exceptionally low sodium levels and extremely high potassium levels. Sodium (Na+) and potassium (K+) are critical for cellular function as many cells rely on a Na/K pump to move molecules across cell walls and for muscles to function properly. Elevated potassium levels—the kind typically seen in Addison's—can induce a fatal heart attack, so an Addisonian crisis is a true emergency.

In addition, Addison's can affect the kidney enzymes, making it look like renal failure. However, once the Addison's is managed with medication, the kidney function returns to normal. Some dogs with Addison's will also present with back pain over the kidneys.

While Addison's is rare, it can happen to any dog. There are breeds at higher risk than others of getting it than others, and it tends to occur more often in females than in males. The breeds at risk:

- Standard poodles

- West Highland White terriers

- Bearded collies

- Rottweilers

- Great Danes

- Newfoundlands

- Portuguese water dogs

- English Springer Spaniels

- German Shorthaired Pointers

- Soft-Coated Wheaten Terriers

- German shepherds

- Labrador Retrievers

- St. Bernards

- Nova Scotia Duck Tolling Retrievers

- Leonbergers

- Welsh Springer Spaniels

In my own personal experience, I see more standard poodles with Addison's than any other breed, but I have seen it in Westies, Labs, and Dachshunds, too. It is still rare compared to Cushing's, but it can also be costly to treat, especially in large dogs. Treatment is aimed at replacing the cortisol in low doses in the form of steroids and replacing the mineralocorticoids with either a monthly injection or pills.

The ACTH stim tests are also used to monitor therapy, especially in the case of treating for Cushing's. The last thing we want to do is inadvertently create Addison's in a dog we're treating for Cushing's! Some of the new medications for Cushing's can alter the function of the adrenal gland so much that this can happen. It is critical to do the follow up tests on the recommended schedule.

Section 12:
Understanding Titers

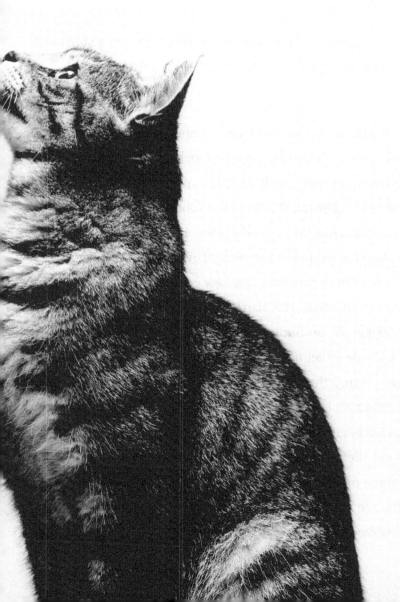

Understanding Titers

First, a few key definitions:

A **titer** is a measurement of the amount or concentration of a substance in a solution and usually refers to the number of antibodies found in blood.

An **antigen** is a substance that can trigger a specific immune response within the host system. It can be organic (such as dust mites, pollen, bacteria, or viruses) or not (such as latex, perfumes, laundry soap, chemical toxins...etc.). The more foreign the substance is to the host, the more likely an immune reaction can take place. Larger molecules are also more likely to trigger an immune response. This is why sometimes when penicillin binds to certain proteins, the new complex can cause allergic reactions in some individuals. It is also how a hapten binding to a platelet can suddenly trigger an autoimmune response to the altered platelet, resulting in a cascade effect of reactions that causes the host system to misidentify and destroy those platelets. This is also why food allergens must be of a certain molecular weight to trigger an allergy. Hydrolyzed proteins that have been altered to be smaller than 13,000 Daltons will not trigger a food allergy because they are too small to do so (this is the basis behind some of the newer hypoallergenic foods for dogs). So, in theory, even though your dog might be allergic to chicken, for example, he can eat hydrolyzed chicken because it can't trigger an allergic reaction.

A **pathogen** is any microorganism (bacteria, virus... etc.) that can cause disease. A pathogen can also be an antigen, but an antigen is not necessarily a pathogen.

The Immune System

The immune system response is an amazingly complex series of reactions in response to a challenge to the host system. Entire textbooks are written on this subject alone, and it is beyond the scope of this manual to explain in detail the intricate workings of immunology and immune system reactions. However, to discuss titers and their interpretation, it helps to know a little about how the immune system recognizes and targets problems. The following is a quick and dirty overview: I wouldn't try to show off your knowledge in a room full of scientists based on this Cliff Notes version of how things work in the immune system!

The function of the immune system is to protect the host from all kinds of antigens. An antigen can be anything that is potentially a threat to the host system. Can you imagine being on duty twenty-four hours a day for the life of your host, constantly processing everything through a massive databank aimed at identifying potential terrorists, and then mobilizing forces to neutralize them before they can wreak havoc? The immune system must have a way of recognizing and **remembering** potential antigens as well as designing extremely specific means of tying up the offending antigen and hustling it out of the way.

The immune system must be flexible and adaptive. It must deal with innumerable potentially dangerous pathogens every day. If the initial defenses are broken (barriers of skin, mucous membranes...etc.) and the first line of defense (the leukocytes and macrophages) is unable to contain the spread of the invasion, then the secondary systems of the immune system are immobilized.

Remember the discussion of lymphocytes in the CBC? I mentioned two basic types based on function, the B cells and the T cells (see Section 2.2 on white blood cell types). B cells form and secrete **antibodies.** These are *matching* counterparts to specific antigens and connect much like a lock and key system. The binding of an antibody to an antigen negates the effect of the antigen. It takes time to create antibodies in response to a new antigen. The lag time between recognition of a new antigen and the creation of significant numbers of antibodies can allow for an overwhelming infection to sweep through the host, especially when the antigens themselves can replicate within the host system like viruses. This is why vaccination is so important and how it prevents disease. Vaccines trigger the antibody production system in a manner that is safer than exposure to the actual infectious agent.

Vaccination

That lag time is why vaccination is so particularly useful in limiting or minimizing the effects of certain diseases. Vaccination allows for a *controlled* exposure of the host to an antigen that has been modified so as not to cause the specific disease in question. The host can then learn to recognize the antigen in the absence of life-threatening illness and thus significantly shorten the lag time before antibody production in the face of exposure to the actual disease.

Say you have a pup that has been vaccinated appropriately against parvo, and it is suddenly challenged by exposure to the real virus. The B cells can immediately start pumping out anti-parvo antibodies because the "order" for the parvo "lock" has previously been processed by the immune system. The "pattern" for the "key" has already been designed, "cut," and programmed into the B cells. This allows the B cells to start producing antibodies in high gear. The binding of an antibody to an antigen makes the entire complex more available for disposal by cells that eat such complexes and digest them. This system is called the **humoral system** because the antibodies circulate in the bloodstream, and because the Greeks referred to blood and bodily fluids as *humors*.

In a typical humoral response, *initial* exposure to the antigen results in a long onset to antibody production (the "lock" must be analyzed, a pattern for the "key" must be designed, and then cut before antibody production can begin). Then, there's a short peak of duration during which the presence of antibodies is detectable in the bloodstream. A second exposure results in a more rapid onset of antibody production but also in a higher and broader peak of duration—so that the response to the second exposure is not only stronger, but the effects last for longer as well.

This is the idea behind booster vaccines for puppies and kittens every 3-4 weeks. Because transfer of maternal antibodies through the first milk can interfere with the puppy's ability to process the antigenic information and because that *interference varies individually for each puppy*, we usually start the initial puppy vaccines at six to eight weeks of age. Then we boost the vaccines every three to four weeks until the puppy is between twelve to sixteen weeks of age. After that, vaccine boosters are recommended one year later and then on differing schedules depending on the duration of immunity and the individual requirement for vaccination.

Stronger immune responses are seen with **modified live vaccines** versus **killed** vaccines. There are reasons why we choose to vaccinate with a killed product at times, however. Rabies is an example of a vaccine that is usually administered as a killed vaccine. A killed vaccine is completely inert and cannot replicate in the host body. You can see why a killed vaccine might be preferable when the risk of developing the actual disease is too great. To stimulate significant immunity for a reasonable period, sometimes vaccines have **adjuvants** added to them. Adjuvants are chemical markers that result in longer-lasting immunity; however, some adjuvants have been linked to adverse effects and are a source of controversy. Vaccine companies continually revise and remodel vaccines to provide the best efficacy while conveying the fewest side effects, but each animal's risk of exposure and the individual needs vary from case to case, as well as with location, lifestyle, and breed sensitivity. Instead of assuming a blanket recommendation to vaccinate for every possible disease under the sun, it is wise to discuss with your veterinarian which vaccines are crucial to protect your pets. Likewise, different localities may have various levels of endemic disease. In our area, we've seen a big increase in the incidence of Lyme disease in the last ten years. Prior to that time, I wasn't a fan of vaccinating for it, in part because the early vaccines had issues with reaction and protection. Now, not only has the incidence changed my recommendations for vaccination, but the vaccines available are superior to the original vaccines. You should discuss with your veterinarian what vaccines your pet may need.

Many veterinary associations have vaccine guidelines that include both **core** vaccines (ones they believe every pet should receive and on what schedule they should receive it) as well as additional vaccines dependent on the individual situation. For example, cats that never go outside or meet other cats are not typically vaccinated for Feline Leukemia. Certain small dog breeds have shown a greater potential for reactions to the

Leptospirosis vaccine, and many vet clinics choose not to vaccinate small dogs with Lepto as a result. In 2015, a new strain of canine influenza entered the U.S., and because no dog here had any immunity to it, the dog flu spread rapidly in kennels and at dog shows. It is now recommended that any dog receiving a Bordetella vaccine to prevent "kennel cough" should also be vaccinated for the canine flu, because the conditions ripe for the spread of respiratory infections are common to both diseases.

Checking Titers Instead of Vaccination

The choice to vaccinate versus check titers on an adult dog is best determined on an individual basis, but the appropriate completion of the puppy series and follow up boosters a year later is considered necessary to attempt to confer a lasting immunity.

If you intend not to vaccinate but to rely on titers the rest of your dog's life, you should complete the puppy series and boost vaccines a year later.

To a certain extent, you are also relying on **herd immunity** to keep your dog safe from infectious disease. Herd immunity is created when a large enough portion of the population has either been vaccinated or has immunity through natural exposure to create resistance to the spread of a particular disease. This level is thought to be at least 80-95% of the population to be protective. It is worth noting that some diseases, such as polio or the measles, never reach herd immunity through natural exposure and have been controlled only through vaccination.

Let's go back to the immune system, and a little more (and more complex!) information to help you understand titers.

You remember we said that lymphocytes come as T or B cells. T lymphocytes secrete substances called *lymphokines* that affect many different cell types and can also act as "killer cells." T cells can also put the brakes on an overactive immune system—when the immune system goes haywire and starts targeting cells that belong to the host system (an *autoimmune response)*. The T cell system can help prevent this in most cases. We refer to the T cell system as **cell-mediated immunity** because of the effects of the lymphokines on other cell types.

The humoral response is effective in dealing with blood-borne antigens but cannot bind to antigens once they are taken up inside a cell (such as a macrophage). Many pathogens replicate *inside* host cells, and thus, they are not available for binding to antibodies. Cell-mediated immunity must then take over the task of destroying the antigen at that point.

On the B cells, the receptor that binds to the circulating antigens is called an **immunoglobulin.** There are five types of immunoglobulins (Ig):

- **IgM** - the precursor for all the other Ig types. It is the first to appear in an antigenic crisis. It forms the majority of the resting B cells.

- **IgG** - produced in greater amounts during the **second** response to an antigenic stimulation. It is the major isotype found in the blood. It will cross the placenta and result in the "passive transfer of antibodies" to the newborn. This is critical for the survival of many species, and failure of passive transfer can result in the death of the newborn.

- **IgD** - when expressed on the same cells as IgM, it activates the resting B cells.

- **IgA** - is found in milk and secretions, in lesser amounts in the bloodstream. IgA deficiencies have been blamed for some food sensitivities.

- **IgE** - is present in low levels but involved in major hypersensitivity (allergic) reactions and in parasitic diseases.

IgM and IgG levels are commonly reported when titers are being measured. High IgM levels can indicate a response to a recent exposure to the antigen in question. High IgG can indicate an older response. Sometimes it is not clear at the time of titer measurement whether you are witnessing an initial response to an antigen or the end of a response (remember the peak of duration and then the drop-off in numbers again?). Sometimes the body retains a positive titer for an exceptionally extended period. It may be necessary to examine the same titers 2-3 weeks after the first analysis. A rapidly rising or falling titer might tell us more than a titer that remains static.

Why do we care about this for the purposes of this discussion?

When we check titers, we are really looking at the amount of immunoglobulin required to react with the antibody in question. A titer is simply a number. It can be "good" when we are seeking a protective response to a vaccine or "bad" when we are looking for a reaction indicating the presence of disease.

A titer is only as reliable as the test itself. For example, some of the first Lyme vaccines could result in a positive titer on testing, which made it difficult to distinguish a true titer from a vaccine response. There are some titers that are notoriously unreliable. In cats, there is a disease called Feline Infectious Peritonitis (FIP). There can be false positives as well as false negatives on the titer testing for this disease. Veterinarians must rely on other information and testing in conjunction with titers when attempting to diagnose this disease.

It might be worth mentioning here that when your vet performs a "snap" test in-house (we mentioned this in Section 7 when talking about tests for heartworm), portions of the test might be checking for antibodies, and portions might be screening for antigens. For example, the combination test for canine heartworms, Lyme, Ehrlichia, and Anaplasmosis screens for heartworm antigens and tick-borne antibodies. If your dog tests positive for heartworms, it is because the antigens were detected in the blood sample, and you can't have heartworm antigens unless heartworms are living inside your dog. However, if your dog tests positive for Lyme, this doesn't necessarily mean your dog *has* Lyme: it means your dog has been exposed and is making antibodies against it. Your dog *might* have Lyme if it is clinically ill at the time of the positive test. Or your dog may simply be showing a positive titer from exposure several years ago. More testing could be necessary before deciding on treatment.

So, when your veterinarian uses a combination heartworm, Ehrlichia, Anaplasmosis, and Lyme snap tests, and your dog test positive for Ehrlichia, should you panic? Not necessarily. Many dogs can have positive snap test results without having the disease itself. These tests are screening tests. Should your dog test positive, you should discuss with your veterinarian if further testing is warranted. It *does* mean that you and your dog live in an area where these diseases are present and that you should be aware and practicing good tick control. But it is not a reason to blindly place all dogs that test positive on a course of antibiotics. The decision to treat should be made on a case-by-case basis.

Not every dog that tests positive for Lyme on a snap test has Lyme. They *are* making Lyme antibodies due to exposure, but they may not actually have Lyme disease. Many of the ancillary "confirmatory" tests are also antibody tests, and it can be hard to interpret whether your dog needs treatment or not. Sometimes the prevalence of tick disease is so common, and your pet has the correct symptoms, so your vet decides to treat rather than pursue expensive titers. Why do we run the snap tests then? Well, if your dog presents with symptoms of Lyme disease, and he tests negative on the snap test, we can take Lyme off the list entirely. A dog will test positive for Lyme before he starts showing clinical signs of the disease. Dogs that have tested positive on the snap tests will often test positive for years.

To make things even more confusing, however; a dog can be ill with Ehrlichia or Anaplasmosis *before* testing positive on these snap tests. Isn't veterinary medicine fun?

So, what do we do when our dogs test positive? There is no easy answer. It depends in part on if we're running these tests because our dogs are ill or if they are turning up as part of routine screening. A blanket call for antibiotics on every dog that tests positive is not the answer. A CBC, chem panel, and urinalysis are usually recommended as follow up testing and running titers or PCR (polymerase chain reaction) tests may be indicated.

A PCR test may be more familiar to you as "DNA" testing. It's a technique that allows even tiny amounts of DNA to be "amplified" to the point of recognition and identification. It's used in forensic medicine as a genetic fingerprint, and it's the basis of paternity testing as well. In diagnostic medicine it is used to detect and identify disease. Because DNA from the organism must be present for any chains to be replicated into a number large enough to identify, a positive test means whatever you're looking for is there—the results can be trusted to be highly accurate. The current recommendation for anything you might want to do PCR testing on is to take a blood sample when the animal first presents with clinical signs and before treatment has been started. You're more likely to get the best results then. The blood can be stored for some time before being sent for testing if it is needed—think of the crimes solved decades later by DNA testing!

Let's look at some examples:

Scooter is a 7-year-old dog with a fever of unknown origin. While working up Scooter's condition, a tick titer panel is run. Scooter's tick panel results come back with a Rocky Mountain Spotted Fever titer (RMSF) result of 1:64. According to this laboratory, this is consistent with exposure to RMSF. But 1:64 is the lowest number at which this titer is considered positive for RMSF. The lab may well recommend a repeat titer check in 2-3 weeks to see if the titer number has risen by 2-3 times the original number. In the meantime, a lack of response to the treatment for RMSF may well change the planned treatment. A low IgM level plus a high IgG level might indicate that this is an old titer response and not a currently active infection.

Misty is an 11-year-old dog with a high fever of unknown origin that is not eating. While the vet is waiting for the results of a tick titer panel, Misty is started on an appropriate dose of doxycycline, and within twenty-four hours, her temperature is normal, and she is eating again. Her RMSF titer comes back as 1:2000. Such a strong titer response in addition to the improvement witnessed by the course of antibiotics supports RMSF as a diagnosis.

Vaccination Versus Titers?

What should you do? What's best for your pet?

The decision to rely on vaccine titers verses periodic vaccination for the adult dog is a personal choice that must be determined between you and your veterinarian. There are many factors involved in this decision-making process, not the least of which includes the local incidence of disease in your area, as well how often your dog interacts with other dogs (competitions, day care, grooming...etc.), the vaccine requirements of facilities in your area, or the type of vaccination used.

In my first year after graduation from vet school, I worked in an extremely rural area where few people vaccinated their dogs. The incidence rate of preventable diseases like parvo and distemper was unbelievable. I diagnosed forty cases of parvo the last month I worked in that area—more than a case per day. This was not an area where I would have felt comfortable recommending replacing annual or semi-annual vaccination with titering. More recently, there was an outbreak of parvo in Alaska that was a particularly nasty strain—even vaccinated dogs were getting it. In the past, certain breeds of dogs (in particular Rottweilers, Dobermans, and Weimaraners) seemed to have trouble assimilating the parvo virus vaccine and required a different vaccination schedule than other breeds. The newer recombinant vaccinations appear to have solved this issue, but I'd have concerns about choosing titers over vaccinations if I had one of these breeds.

On the other hand, if I see a dog develop an autoimmune reaction shortly after receiving its assortment of annual vaccines, I recommend that it never be vaccinated ever again for anything but rabies, and I will write a letter exempting it from vaccination for the purposes of boarding or hospitalization. Keep in mind when travelling that acceptance of titers in lieu of vaccine certificates, while growing, is not universal. Make sure that if you intend to kennel your dog at your point of destination that you confirm in advance that a titer will be accepted.

Vaccine protocols and recommendations change over time. As I've said before, Lyme disease wasn't an issue in our area until about ten years ago. As recent studies are performed and new vaccines are developed, and new diseases arise, what may have been standard in the past might be revised in the light of new information. More clinics are moving away from the "one size fits all" mentality of vaccination and are structuring protocols around the individual pet. This is definitely a conversation for you to have with your veterinarian based on your pet's needs.

Section 13:

Case Studies

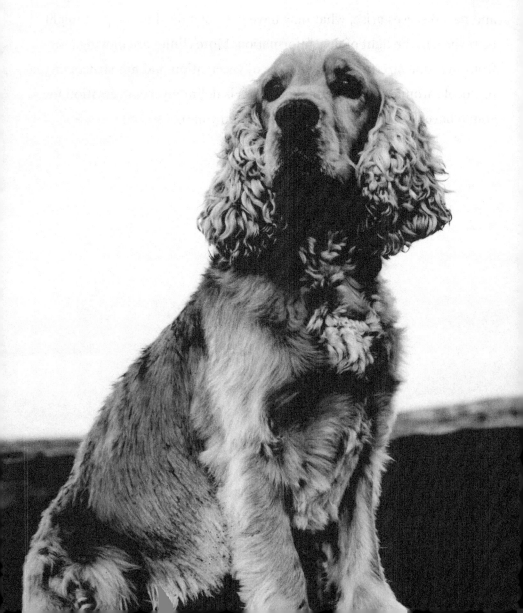

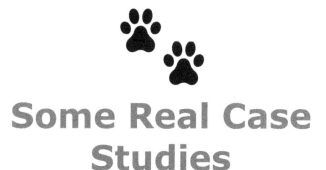

Some Real Case Studies

Most of the examples that I have presented thus far have been simplified cases that highlight one or two problems in the lab work. Here, I have included a few real-life cases for comparison to show some of the considerations that can affect interpretation of the lab work results.

Real Case #1 – Charlie, 11-year-old, neutered male Cocker Spaniel

Charlie is an 11-year-old neutered male cocker spaniel. Doctors call this description of Charlie (age, sex, breed) a **signalment** and it standardizes the way veterinarians describe cases to one another. The signalment can be particularly important to determining what is wrong with our patient. For instance, a spayed female dog is highly unlikely to have a pyometra, and as such, this would not be on the rule out list if she presented for illness. The signalment gives the who/what/where of the case. Think Colonel Mustard in the library with the candlestick.

Charlie presents (another veterinary term, meaning "When Charlie walked in my exam room door…") with a 2-3 day history of vomiting and refusal to eat (**anorexia**). On physical exam, Charlie has lost four pounds since his last documented weight six months previously. He is dehydrated; his skin over his shoulders is slow to slide back into place when lifted and released. His gums are sticky rather than slick and moist. He is depressed (lacked energy or interest in surroundings) and is salivating (a sign of nausea).

Charlie's bloodwork is run on an in-house Idexx machine and looks like this:

CBC	Results		Reference Range
HCT	30.5 %	(LOW)	37-55

CBC	Results		Reference Range
HCB	10.7 g/dl	(LOW)	12-16
WBC	10.5 10⁹/L		6-16.9
NEUT	84 10⁹/L		2.8-10.5
EOS	0.9 10⁹/L		0.5-1.5
Lymphocyte/monocyte ratio (L/M)	1.2 10⁹/L		1.1-6.5
PLT	386 10⁹/L		175-500
Reticulocytes	0.3%		

On this Idexx machine, lymphocyte and monocyte numbers are presented as a ratio instead of the actual individual numbers. As such, the machine in question is not sensitive enough to distinguish bands from mature neutrophils. The results of this CBC indicate that Charlie is mildly anemic and that his anemia does not appear to be regenerative (as he does not have a strong reticulocyte response).

His chemistry profile:

Chemistry	Results		Reference Range
ALB	2.95 g/dl		2.7-3.8
ALKP	71 U/L		23-212
ALT	64 U/L		10-100
AMYL	outside analyzer range		500-1500
BUN	110.8 mg/dl	(HIGH)	7-27
CHOL	219 mg/dl		110-320
CREAT	3.4 mg/dl	(HIGH)	0.5-1.8
GLU	142.7 mg/dl		77-125
CA	7.66 mg/dl		7.9-12
PHOS	>16 mg/dl	(HIGH)	2.5-6.8
TBILI	0.26 mg/dl		0-0.9

Chemistry	Results	Reference Range
TP	6.94 g/dl	5.2-8.2
GLOB	3.99 g/dl	2.5-4.5

A dog with dehydration and is vomiting with these blood values could be showing signs of both pancreatitis and kidney failure. Because this Idexx machine can only run twelve assays at a time and because the amylase levels are higher than the machine was able to determine, separate amylase and lipase levels were sent to an independent laboratory. Today, a tableside canine lipase test might be run instead.

Antech Lab results:

AMYL	2545 U/L (HIGH)	290-1125
LIPA	451 U/L	77-695

Note: notice how the amylase reference range for normal at the Antech lab is different from the Idexx reference range. **You must always compare test results with the reference range provided by the laboratory system on which the test was performed.**

Because the lipase levels are normal despite amylase elevations, pancreatitis is not likely. The reason for the markedly elevated amylase levels is a decreased kidney filtration rate, which is altering the rate at which amylase is cleared from the body. Charlie's primary problem would appear to be chronic kidney failure. Why chronic kidney failure and not acute?

- Charlie has lost significant weight in the last six months

- Charlie has a mild non-regenerative anemia (remember erythropoietin?)

- In addition to the elevated BUN and creatinine levels, Charlie also has increased phosphorous levels (which tends to happen with more chronic kidney disease)

Charlie responds well to a three-day course of IV fluid therapy, which reduces his BUN and creatinine levels and improves his kidney filtration rate. His BUN and creatinine levels remain above normal but are less than at his initial presentation. He is placed on the Hill's Prescription Diet k/d for chronic kidney dysfunction. This diet is a low protein/phosphorus diet that is also high in fat to help maintain body weight. Chronic renal failure (CRF) is a progressive disease process. Diet management improves Charlie's quality of life and reduces the work that his kidneys had to perform to process his food, but over the period of a year, his kidney function continues to deteriorate, and his people opt to have him euthanized.

Ironically, another cocker spaniel came in the same week, also in kidney failure. Crystal is a 6-year-old spayed female cocker spaniel that had gotten into her owner's luggage and eaten some ibuprofen. Her lab work looks almost identical to Charlie's with some notable exceptions: she is not anemic, and she does not have the grossly elevated phosphorus levels. There is no history of weight loss, either. Crystal has **acute renal failure.** She receives the same essential treatment as Charlie, but her blood values return to normal with treatment and remain that way for the next several years. It will be interesting to see if Crystal's kidney function remains normal throughout her life. Such a toxic insult to the kidneys is likely to affect her kidney health as she ages.

Real Case #2 – Marlboro, 7-year-old neutered male Beagle

Marlboro is a 7-year-old neutered male beagle. He presents with a history of decreased energy and periodic weakness. His owner thinks he might be having mild seizures.

On physical examination, Marlboro has a Grade 3/6 heart murmur, meaning on a scale of 1 to 6, his murmur was a Grade 3. Heart sounds are usually the result of the valves closing during the normal heartbeat cycle. "Leaky" valves allow a backwash of blood through the valve creating the sound of the murmur. Heart murmurs are graded as to the degree of loudness and intensity on a scale from 1 to 6, with 6 being the loudest. Sometimes, Roman numerals are used to characterize the murmur grade, but the scale is the same. Marlboro has extremely pale mucus membranes—his gums are very pale, almost white in appearance instead of a healthy pink.

Marlboro's lab results (performed on an in-house Idexx machine):

CBC	Results		Reference Range
HCT	9.5%	(LOW)	37-55
HCB	3.2 g/dl	(LOW)	12-16
WBC	5.9 10⁹/L		6-16.9

CBC	Results		Reference Range
NEUT	4.2 10⁹/L		2.8-10.5
EOS	0 10⁹/L		0.5-1.5
Lymph/mono ratio (L/M)	1.7 10⁹/L		1.1-6.5
PLT	855 10⁹/L	(HIGH)	175-500
Reticulocytes	0		

Marlboro's chemistry profile is all completely within normal limits. A clotting profile was sent to Antech Laboratories to rule out a bleeding disorder, and those test results are also completely within normal limits.

First, Marlboro is in serious trouble here. He is severely anemic and with a hematocrit of less than 12%. He needs a blood transfusion. As the heart murmur was a new physical exam finding, it is entirely possible that the murmur is the result of the extreme thinness of his blood creating more turbulence as it passes through the heart—thus creating the *sound* of a leaky heart valve. If this is the case, the murmur will resolve once the HCT is back in the normal range.

There is no evidence of regeneration as shown by the absence of reticulocytes. Non-regenerative anemias are more serious because it usually means something is preventing the bone marrow from recognizing or responding to the crisis. Because his chemistry profile is normal (no icterus, no elevated bilirubin or ALT levels) there is no indication that this is a hemolytic anemia. It may still be an immune-mediated problem, but it is unlikely that the red cells are being destroyed at an abnormal rate because there are no by-products of that destruction showing up in the lab work. Note the elevated platelet count. Although in general, elevated platelet counts are not of great concern in the dog, the magnitude of the elevation and the absence of regeneration makes me question what is going on in the bone marrow. It looks like at least something unusual to say the least.

Marlboro receives a blood transfusion. This brings his HCT up to 15% and improves his energy and appetite. It's amazing how much improved Marlboro is with just a slight boost in his HCT. He's referred on an emergency basis to a specialty practice for a bone marrow aspirate.

The bone marrow aspirate reveals a yucky "myeloproliferative infiltrate." That was the closest description we could get of this unknown substance that was filling his bone marrow and replacing the healthy tissue. This is bad news. Your bone marrow is the nursery for all your red and white blood cells. Once Marlboro's circulating cells died off from old age, they could not be replaced. Eventually, even with repeated transfusions, Marlboro would die if the disease process could not be halted.

Marlboro is started on immunosuppressive doses of prednisone, as well as a stomach protecting medication to help prevent ulcers. Of equal concern is the possibility that therapy will make him susceptible to infection, and he would not be able to respond with increased white cell production. Marlboro comes in for a CBC every two weeks while undergoing chemotherapy. It takes four weeks before his HCT begins to improve at all, but by week six on prednisone, his HCT is 40%.

Marlboro feels great and is beginning to get as fat as a little pig (one of the side effects of steroids), so we begin the slow process of weaning him off medication. We reduce his prednisone dose by 25% every four weeks. It takes eight months, but Marlboro is weaned off medication entirely and comes in for periodic testing at this point. Not knowing exactly what triggered the underlying problem or indeed exactly what the underlying condition was, it is difficult to say whether it will recur. Marlboro had not been vaccinated for a least 3 years prior to his illness. Because he does have some sort of autoimmune disease condition, however; at this time, he only receives a rabies vaccine once every 3 years as required by state law.

Real Case #3 – Ginger, 6-year-old spayed female Australian Shepherd

Ginger is a 6-year-old spayed female Australian Shepherd. At 60 pounds, she is approximately 20 pounds overweight. She presents late on a Friday afternoon in a state of collapse after a history of taking a long walk in 100-degree weather. On arrival at the vet clinic, her body temperature is 106.6 degrees.

Vet #1 stabilizes Ginger by treating her for shock and heatstroke, starting her on an IV fluid drip and administering a cooling bath. Heatstroke can result in multi-system organ failure because of the heat stress and shock.

Ginger's initial bloodwork results (abbreviated):

CBC	Results		Reference Range
HCT	56.6	(HIGH)	37-55
HCB	19.8 g/dl	(HIGH)	12-16
WBC	20 10⁹/L	(HIGH)	6-16.9
EOS	0 10⁹/L		0.5-1.5

CBC	Results		Reference Range
Lymph/mono ratio (L/M)	1.8 10^9/L		1.1-6.5
PLT	56 10^9/L	(LOW)	175-500
Reticulocytes	0		

Chemistry profile:

Chemistry	Results		Reference Range
ALB	4.05 g/dl	(HIGH)	2.7-3.8
ALKP	214 U/L	(HIGH)	23-212
ALT	Outside analyzer range		10-100
AMYL	1369 U/L		500-1500

Chemistry	Results		Reference Range
BUN	81.3 mg/dl	(HIGH)	7-27
CHOL	520 mg/dl	(HIGH)	110-320
CREAT	5.59 mg/dl	(HIGH)	0.5-1.8
GLU	105.2 mg/dl		77-125
CA	8.77 mg/dl		7.9-12
PHOS	12.6 mg/dl	(HIGH)	2.5-6.8
TBILI	0.84/dl		0-0.9
TP	5.94 g/dl		5.2-8.2
GLOB	3.45 g/dl		2.5-4.5

Electrolytes are within normal limits.

Ginger's temperature can only be reduced to 104 degrees through treatment. Ginger is in multi-system organ failure, possibly because of the heatstroke. The concentration of her PCV values and elevated white cell count are attributed to the state of shock that she is in. Her decreased platelet numbers are possibly due to abnormally rapid clotting of blood, which is not unusual in heatstroke victims. Ginger is started on a broad-spectrum antibiotic and transferred to the local animal emergency clinic for further care during the weekend. Despite the elevated phosphorus levels, there is no history of weight loss or anemia, making it less likely that her kidney troubles are chronic and more likely they are part of the overall sudden illness.

Over the weekend, Ginger remains on IV fluids. Her temperature drops to 103.7 but does not return to normal. This makes heatstroke as the cause of the elevated temperature less likely now. Vet #2 continues supportive care and decides to change antibiotics after 12 hours with no response on the original medication. Vet #3 cares for Ginger the following day and adds another antibiotic to what she is currently taking as Ginger continues to run a fever and refuses to eat. Radiographs and ultrasound were performed of the chest and abdomen; no abnormalities are found. Vet #4 inherits Ginger on Monday when she is referred to the original vet's office after the weekend.

This no longer appears to be a simple case of heatstroke. While multi-system organ failure is a potential complication of heatstroke, Ginger received prompt attention and aggressive treatment for her clinical signs. Prolonged elevation of temperature is not usually seen with heatstroke once treatment has begun. Vet #4 decides to repeat the lab work to check Ginger's progress.

Ginger's lab work after 3 days of antibiotics and IV fluids (performed on an Idexx machine):

CBC	Results		Reference Range
HCT	39%		37-55
HCB	14.3 g/dl		12-16
WBC	13.2 10⁹/L		6-16.9
NEUT	12.0 10⁹/L		2.8-10.5
EOS	0 10⁹/L		0.5-1.5
Lymph/mono ratio (L/M)	1.2 10⁹/L		1.1-6.5
PLT	86 10⁹/L	(LOW)	175-500
Reticulocytes			0

Whoa! While much of the CBC has improved (by correcting the fluid abnormalities associated with shock), that platelet count is still exceptionally low. It has improved a little, but it still bears close monitoring.

Chemistry profile:

Chemistry	Results		Reference Range
ALB	2.94 g/dl		2.7-3.8
ALKP	308 U/L	(HIGH)	23-212
ALT	614 U/L	(HIGH)	10-100
AMYL	1368 U/L		500-1500
BUN	82.0 mg/dl	(HIGH)	7-27
CHOL	28 mg/dl		110-320
CREAT	4.08 mg/dl	(HIGH)	0.5-1.8
GLU	105.2 mg/dl		77-125
CA	8.77 mg/dl		7.9-12
PHOS	5.31 mg/dl		2.5-6.8

Chemistry	Results		Reference Range
TBILI	2.44 mg/dl	(HIGH)	0-0.9
TP	6.37 g/dl		5.2-8.2
GLOB	3.43 g/dl		2.5-4.5

Electrolytes:

Na: 167 mmol/L (HIGH)	144-160
K: 2.75 mmol/L (LOW)	3.5-5.8
Cl: 117 mmol/L	109-122

Urinalysis:

SpGr 1.010 (LOW)	1.040 and above
Protein: + +	0 to trace amounts

PH 5	5-6.5
Bilirubin (elevated)	trace amounts in normal urine

The rest of the urinalysis is within normal limits, no bacteria or white cells noted on sediment.

Well, there has scarcely been any improvement at all. While the ALT is at least on the scale again, the ALKP has increased. Worse, so has the total bilirubin. Just another few points on the T bili, and Ginger will be turning visibly icteric to the eye—her mucous membranes will become as yellow as a ripe banana (remember, excess bilirubin will spill over into the urine, before it rises in the blood).

Her kidney function has not really improved either: although the phosphorous is down, her BUN and creatinine are hardly changed at all. This is very discouraging for three days of ICU care, especially when we are no closer to understanding what is wrong with Ginger in the first place. Her abnormal electrolyte levels could be due to the use of a potassium-poor IV fluid solution or due to her lack of eating. The urine results are consistent with her kidney dysfunction and show no signs of infection. Officially, Ginger is considered to have **fever of unknown origin (FUO).** Ginger continues to be very depressed and refuses to eat.

FUO can be exceedingly difficult to diagnose and treat. At this point, Ginger has been on three different antibiotics, and her CBC does not support signs of infection, but something is causing the fever. Something is suppressing her platelet count. Something is damaging her liver and kidney function. Many rickettsial diseases spread by ticks can have this kind of widespread effect on the body, but one of the antibiotics chosen by the emergency clinic was doxycycline, which is usually highly effective against these organisms. Ginger has shown no response to this medication.

It should be noted that sometimes doxycycline can cause liver enzymes to elevate, but there are usually no clinical symptoms associated with this type of elevation.

Performing a liver or kidney biopsy on Ginger is contraindicated with the low platelet count—serious, even fatal bleeding could result at the biopsy site. Radiographs and ultrasound were non-diagnostic. A blood culture is costly and time-consuming, and with Ginger's antibiotic history, it is most likely to fail to garner positive results. In fact, although given in an honest attempt to treat Ginger on an emergency basis, the antibiotic history now makes further diagnostics a bit problematic. We don't know what Ginger's urine looked like before therapy—there was no time to get a sample before stabilization and transfer. Blood cultures can take up to a week to get results and are seldom needed; changing antibiotics when she failed to improve was appropriate. But now what? We need to somehow determine the cause of the fever and treat it, hoping that the organ failure will respond as well.

What happens is that Ginger's owners, distraught at the severity of her illness, the cost of continued therapy, and the increasingly dim prognosis for recovery, opt to have her euthanized. They set up a time to visit her late in the day to say their goodbyes and have the euthanasia performed. Vet #4 in the meantime, looks over the treatment history for Ginger over the last few days.

What she sees is that initially Ginger has been given a good broad-spectrum antibiotic that was effective against many gram-positive and gram-negative organisms. Antibiotic number two was effective against rickettsial organisms. Antibiotic number three was effective against many organisms that have become resistant to the common antibiotics and using it in conjunction with antibiotic number two allows for a wide range of activity. However, Vet #4 realizes that of all the choices administered so far, none of these medications would be effective against **anaerobic** organisms—those bacteria that live deep in the tissues and survive in low oxygen atmospheres. Sometimes in veterinary medicine, we refer to a **four-quad approach** to antibiotic coverage, especially when the infectious agent has not been identified. This is shorthand for a four-quadrant approach—the four quadrants being gram-negative, gram-positive, aerobic, and anaerobic organisms. In Ginger's case, the anaerobic component had not yet been addressed with an antibiotic trial.

A good anaerobic antibiotic is available in the hospital, but it is contraindicated for use in dogs with liver failure because of potential serious side effects. Vet #4 looks at her watch and decides that since Ginger is scheduled to be euthanized in a few hours anyway, what difference would it make? She administers a dose of that antibiotic. Two hours later, Ginger is up on her feet, barking, and looking for food. Her temperature is normal. At this point, her owners are persuaded to give her additional time on IV fluids and the new medication.

Ginger continues to improve and is discharged on the fourth antibiotic. Her lab results three weeks later:

- CBC completely within normal limits. Her platelet count was
  472×10^3

- Chemistry panel completely within normal limits EXCEPT cholesterol 483.6

Because of the persistent elevation of the cholesterol, Ginger is tested for hypothyroidism. She proves to be hypothyroid, and after starting supplementation, she drops fifteen pounds.

We never did determine what caused Ginger's illness. Her successful treatment was not the result of careful diagnostic testing—in fact, it flew in the face of recommended therapy for a dog in her condition. The goals of medicine sometimes get constrained between what should be done, has been done, and can be done. Her hypothyroidism may have predisposed her to some infectious agent but was not the ultimate cause of illness. Four years later, she is still doing well with no apparent aftereffects of her original illness.

Summary

Hopefully, you will be in a better position now to understand the value as well as the limitations of certain lab tests. I think you can see why there might be ambiguity in interpreting some bloodwork results. It is my sincerest hope that this information will help you converse with your veterinarian about specific laboratory findings on your pets and place you in a better position to make certain decisions about the diagnosis, treatment, and general well-being of your beloved family member. Don't be afraid to ask questions. Then run home and read some more in this book!

Glossary of Terms

Acute: any set of symptoms or a condition that appears suddenly in onset without previous warning or history.

Alanine transferase: (ALT) one of the liver enzymes released by the death of liver cells and, thus, a sensitive indicator of a current or ongoing liver problem.

Albumin: largest protein that circulates in the blood stream, responsible in part for maintaining the integrity of the blood vessels through **oncotic** pressure.

Alkaline phosphatase: (ALKP) one of the blood enzymes used to assess liver function. Produced by the liver but also has other sources in the body including the bones. Can be "activated" by certain medications and so is not a specific indicator of liver health.

Amylase: an enzyme produced by the pancreas and the salivary glands to aid in digestion. Elevations can indicate pancreatitis (see **pancreatitis**) or kidney disease.

Anaphylactic shock: a life-threatening condition in which some reaction (usually allergic) triggers a massive breakdown of mast cells within the body, releasing huge volumes of histamines and other chemicals into the blood stream. Can result in rapid death without warning.

Anemia: a reduction in the number of red cells or hemoglobin levels below normal.

Anion: a negatively charged ion. Will attract and bond to positively charged ions to form salts (see **cation**).

Anorexia: simply stated, a refusal to eat food. Can occur for a wide variety of reasons.

Antigen: substance capable of triggering a specific immune response within the host system.

Antibodies: matching counterparts to antigens created specifically by the body to negate the effects of that antigen.

Ascites: the development of fluid freely collecting within the abdomen.

Atrophy: a state whereby a cell, organ, or living system withers away and dies, usually from lack of energy, blood supply, or nervous input.

Attrition: term used to refer to the natural wear, aging, and death of physiological subjects. Can be used to describe wear patterns and loss of teeth, dying off cells or populations of animals.

Autoimmune: a condition whereby the immune system of the patient inappropriately targets cells or tissue that belong to that patient as a foreign invader and actively begin destroying that matter.

Azotemia: an elevation of urea levels in the bloodstream (see BUN)

Band cells: immature neutrophils that are being released by the bone marrow before maturation, usually in response to an overwhelming infection. Large elevations in band cell counts indicate serious, life-threatening infection.

Basophils: one of the several types of white cells. Circulates in sparse numbers and is rarely identified in disease conditions.

Benign: term used to describe the behavior and characteristics of tumor or disease condition that is not harmful and carries a good prognosis.

Bilirubin: originates inside red blood cells and certain macrophages. Converted to bile by the liver. Elevated levels in the blood leads to **icterus (see icterus, see jaundice).**

Bilirubinemia: state whereby elevated levels of bilirubin are measurable in the bloodstream.

Bilirubinuria: state whereby excess bilirubin is processed through the kidneys and out the urine as waste in elevated levels.

Blood sugar: another term for glucose. A simple sugar measured in the blood stream. The only means of energy suitable to sustain normal brain function. The body converts most ingested sugars into this form. (See **glucose**)

BUN: (Blood Urea Nitrogen, Urea Nitrogen) a by-product of protein metabolism produced by the liver and removed from the body by the kidneys. Elevated BUN levels are a state also known as **azotemia.**

Cachexia: an abnormal state of metabolism in which energy demands exceed available energy and the body enters a state of rapid wasting, resulting in extreme muscle and tissue loss. Can be seen in advanced stages of heart disease and some forms of cancer or metabolic imbalance.

Cation: a positively charged ion that will attract and bond to negatively charged ions (see **anion)** to form salts.

Cell-mediated immunity: the kind of immunity conferred by the secretions of certain chemicals (see **lymphokines)** by specialized cells that have effects on other cells within the host system.

Chemistry panel (serum chemistry panel, chem panel): a measurement of certain enzymes in the blood sample (serum) of a particular patient or subject. Varies between laboratories as to normal ranges and specific tests included in the screen.

Complete cell count (CBC): an accounting of the total numbers of red and white cells within a blood sample of a particular subject or patient. If the white cell numbers are also counted individually according to type, this is considered a **differential.**

Centrifugation: a method of concentrating cells numbers normally suspended in a fluid sample by spinning the sample at high speeds to separate the fluid component from the cellular component.

Chloride: (CL-) one of the electrolytes commonly measured; an anion that will bond to a cation.

Cholestasis: the development of bile products in elevated levels in the blood stream.

Colitis: an inflammation of the large bowel characterized by straining to defecate (see **tenesmus**) and the production of small, loose stools with or without accompanying mucus or frank blood.

Cornea: the clear, shiny surface of the eye.

Cortisol: hormone secreted by the adrenal glands in response to stresses. Necessary in small quantities to support life functions.

Creatinine: substance produced in small quantities by the body. Direct correlation to kidney filtration rate and therefore used to assess kidney function.

Cystocentesis: method of collecting urine in a sterile fashion by inserting a needle through the body wall and directly into the bladder.

Differential: an accounting of the numbers of white cells in each blood sample, grouped according to white cell type and reported in relative proportion to each other. **(See CBC).**

Eclampsia: a condition in which circulating levels of calcium drop dangerously low, resulting in uncontrollable muscle contractions (see **tetany**).

Edema: the development of fluid within the tissues or lungs.

Endocrine: part of the body system that secretes hormones to control important bodily functions and balances.

Electrolytes: certain salts that circulate within the blood supply and operate on the cellular level to conduct energy. They are vital to the normal operation of cell function, including muscle contraction and the transport of materials in an out across cell membranes.

Emaciation: term used to describe extreme thinness, usually due to disease or starvation.

Eosinophils: one of the types of white cells usually identified with parasitic or allergic conditions.

Erythropoietin: a natural hormone produced by the kidneys that stimulates red cell production by the bone marrow. Can be depressed in advanced kidney disease, resulting in chronic anemia. Available for medical use as a red cell production stimulate for patients with advanced kidney disease or undergoing chemotherapy that effects bone marrow function.

Exocrine: part of the body system that secretes a hormone or enzyme through a duct system.

Familial: a group of animals that are related. A disease condition that appears in a higher incidence among related dogs than between non-related dogs is considered to have a familial basis. Unless test breedings are performed to confirm transfer of this genetic tendency, it is not considered an inherited trait.

Febrile: a state of having an elevated body temperature or fever

Fever of Unknown Origin (FUO): phrase used to describe a condition in which the patient is running a fever and the cause has not or cannot be determined.

Frank blood: term used to describe the loss of fresh (red) blood into a substance as opposed to melena which is digested blood (black).

Glomerular nephritis: a progressive destruction of the main functional unit of the kidney. The most common form of kidney dysfunction in the dog. Sometimes referred to as **nephritis** for short.

Glomerulus: one of the parts of the basic unit of filtration within the kidney.

Glucose: a simple sugar necessary to normal brain function and a readily accessible form of energy. Typically referred to as "blood glucose" (see **blood sugar).**

Glucosuria: the presence of glucose in the urine.

Hematocrit: a means of assessing red cell numbers to determine if a patient is anemic. Term derives from device used to concentrate the red cell numbers and measure their volume against a grid that correlates to certain percentages. This term can be exchanged equally for **PCV (see packed cell volume).**

Hemoconcentration: condition in which the fluid portion of the blood is severely depleted, resulting in a relative increase in the proportion of red cells on the CBC. Red cell numbers in the 6-8% concentration range can be life-threatening (see **hemorrhagic gastroenteritis).**

Hemorrhagic gastroenteritis (HGE): is a life-threatening medical condition in which large volumes of fluid are being dumped into the gastrointestinal tract that is concurrently sloughing (losing due to death of cells) large amounts of mucosa (absorptive surface). It results in a measurement of red cell counts above normal on a CBC (**hemoconcentration**).

Humoral immunity: the type of immunity conferred by the production of antibodies that circulate in the bloodstream (see **antibodies**).

Hyperadrenocorticism: (Cushing's disease) abnormally elevated levels of cortisol in the blood stream, usually as the result of a tumor secreting that hormone.

Hypoadrenocorticism: (Addison's disease) life-threatening condition whereby the body is incapable of secreting enough cortisol and other hormones necessary to maintain normal electrolyte balance within the body.

Hyperglycemia: persistently elevated levels of blood sugar; usually associated with diabetes.

Hypoglycemia: exceptionally low levels of blood sugar.

Icterus: term that is interchangeable with older term **jaundice**. A medical condition where the blood bilirubin levels (**bilirubinemia**) has risen to such an extent that the whites of the eyes and the mucus membranes are visibly turning yellow.

Idiopathic: term meaning the origin or cause is unknown.

Immunoglobulin: a receptor in the B cell lymphocytes that binds to specific antigens.

Ischemia: a condition where a part of the body has been severely deprived of its normal blood flow, resulting in tissue damage and death.

Jaundice: see icterus. Jaundice is the human term versus the animal one, more people have heard of it than icterus.

Keratoconjunctivitis sicca: (KSC, "dry eye") condition in which tear production is below normal for a wide variety of reasons, resulting in abnormal changes to the cornea.

Ketoacidosis: a state in which the pH of the blood becomes too acidic due to the presence of large numbers of ketones.

Ketones: (ketone bodies) a by-product of protein and fat metabolism. Seen in conditions of rapid weight-loss such as starvation and in certain states of diabetes.

Larval migrans: condition in which a parasite (usually not normal to the infected host) migrates abnormally through the host tissues to carry out its life cycle.

Left shift: term used to describe an elevation in band cells (see **band cells)** while the overall number of neutrophils are normal or decreased.

Leptospirosis: an infectious disease seen in dogs that can cause acute liver and kidney failure.

Leukemia: a disease condition characterized by a grossly elevated white cell count, or when the white cells themselves are grossly abnormal in shape.

Leukemoid reaction: white cell numbers exceeding 50,000 to 100,000 in a blood sample.

Lipase: one of the enzymes secreted by the pancreas to aid in digestion. Elevations usually indicate pancreatitis (see **pancreatitis**).

Lymphocytes: one of the types of white cells. Second line of defense. Numbers greatest in more chronic disease states. Divided into two types

(B and T cells), which have distinct roles within the immune system. Responsible for creating antibodies.

Lymphokines: specialized chemicals produced by the T-lymphocytes that effect other cells in the immune defense system.

Macrophages: large white cells that remove dying and dead debris from the living system.

Malignant: term used to describe the behavior and characteristics of a deadly tumor or disease process and carries a poor prognosis.

Mast cells: a type of inflammatory cell that contains large amounts of histamine and other chemicals inside granules within the cell. Can be associated with anaphylactic shock (see **anaphylactic shock**) and certain types of skin tumors.

Melena: black, tar-like feces that indicate the presence of digested blood; an indication of gastrointestinal bleeding (stomach ulcers, cancer...etc.).

Metastasis: the spread of a malignant tumor through the blood or lymphatic systems to set up growth and production in sites more distant from the original growth.

Minimum database (MDB): a medical term used to refer to a grouping of medical tests designed to broadly screen for health issues in a particular patient or subject. Varies to some degree concerning species and personal preferences. Usually taken to mean a CBC, serum chemistry panel, urinalysis, fecal analysis, and heartworm test for most dogs.

Monocytes: a type of white cell that circulates briefly in the blood stream before maturing into macrophages (see **macrophages).**

Morphology (cell): a description of the visible appearance of cell types.

Motile: term used to describe bacteria or protozoan life forms that can self-propel or swim in the host environment.

Neoplasia: another term for cancer.

Nephritis: inflammation of the nephrons of the kidney, short for **glomerular nephritis**.

Nephron: in conjunction with the glomerulus, makes up the main functional unit of the kidney (see also **glomerulus, glomerular nephritis).**

Nephropathy: a disease condition related to the kidneys.

Nephrotic syndrome: condition in which normal kidney architecture is replaced by abnormal proteins. Characterized by markedly elevated urine protein levels and elevated fat levels in the blood and urine, as well as peripheral limb edema.

Neutrophils: primary white cell that fights disease. Constitutes the first line of defense and therefore make up the highest proportion of white cell numbers.

Nucleated red blood cells: immature red blood cells that have been released early from the bone marrow before completing maturation, usually in response to excessive need in an anemic patient. **(Also called reticulocytes).**

Occult: term used to describe an infection that has no outward symptoms, most often used to describe a heartworm infection in which there are no circulating microfilaria in the bloodstream.

Ocular: related to the eye

Oncotic pressure: the pressure induced by the presence of molecules within a fluid that acts as a counterbalance to the pressure exerted by the capillaries.

Operculum: a small "trapdoor" on the surface of a parasite egg that opens to release its contents.

Otitis: an infection or inflammation of the ear.

Packed cell volume (PCV): a means of measuring the relative volume of red cells in each blood sample to determine if a patient is anemic. Reported as a percentage of the red cells relative to the plasma within a blood sample after centrifugation.

Pancreatitis: an inflammation of the pancreas, usually in response to infection or the consumption of fatty foods leading to the self-digestion of that organ through an over-production of digestive enzymes.

Panleukopenia: an across the board decrease of all the white cell numbers, due to either infection or suppression of the bone marrow.

Peripheral: pertaining to the extremities; can be used to describe the ears, legs, tail...etc.

pH: a measure of the relative acidity or alkaline nature of a body of fluid. Neutral pH is 7.0. Acidic fluids are less than 7.0 in pH. Alkaline fluids are greater than 7.0.

Platelets: produced by the bone marrow and aid in clotting of the blood. Most common abnormalities of platelet function are autoimmune thrombocytopenia and Von Willebrand's disease. (See **thrombocytes**)

Potassium: (K+) an electrolyte commonly measured in the bloodstream. Responsible for many essential functions on a cellular level. Tolerated in a very narrow range within the living system. Abnormalities of potassium levels can be life-threatening.

Propylene glycol: a sugary sweet substance that is a food additive in many dog foods and is enough chemically related to antifreeze (ethylene glycol) that it can result in a positive reaction on an antifreeze test.

Pyelonephritis: an infection of the kidneys.

Renal: term given to the kidney and is interchangeable with that word.

Resorbed: a term used to describe the body's ability to slowly break down dead and dying material and re-assimilate it into the host system over time.

Reticulocytes: immature red blood cells released early from the bone marrow, usually in response to anemia. Also known as **nucleated red blood cells.**

Septicemia: a generalized (systemic) infection of microorganisms or toxins in the bloodstream.

Signalment: a standardized term used to describe baseline information about a patient, such as age, sex, and breed.

Sodium: (NA+) an important electrolyte measured in the blood stream. Must be kept in balance with potassium levels for the normal function of cells. Abnormalities of sodium levels can be life-threatening.

Spherocytes: an abnormal red blood cell seen in cases of autoimmune hemolytic anemia.

Splenic contraction: condition in which the spleen of an excited animal contracts during the blood collection procedure, suddenly dumping part of its reservoir of blood into the main artery/venous system. This results in mild to moderate artificial elevation of certain cell numbers on a CBC (including red cells, white cells, and platelets) and must be factored in when assessing the CBC.

Tenesmus: term to describe the condition of straining to defecate (see colitis).

Tetany: a condition in which the muscle uncontrollably contracts. Certain poisons and metabolic conditions can result in tetanic seizures or contractions. The condition of tetanus is when the muscles are not able to relax due to the presence of a toxin paralyzing them in the contracted state.

Thrombocytes (platelets): produced by the bone marrow and aid in clotting of the blood. Most common abnormalities of platelet function are autoimmune thrombocytopenia and Von Willebrand's disease.

Thyroid: a gland that produces thyroid hormone. Thyroid hormone is responsible for controlling metabolic rate.

Translocation: a shift from the blood circulation into the cellss of various substances, rendering them unavailable for use at that time.

Translocation can result in apparent deficiencies that must not be over-corrected once the condition that triggered the translocation (shock, acidosis...etc.) has been corrected.

Urine Specific gravity: a means of measuring the kidney's ability to concentrate urine normally.

Uveitis: an infection within the globe of the eye.

References

American Chemical Society. (2007). *Cat Disease Linked to Flame Retardants in Furniture and to Pet Food.* ScienceDaily. https://www.sciencedaily.com/releases/2007/08/070815122354. htm

American Society of Nephrology (ASN). (2014). *Toxin in Seafood Causes Kidney Damage in Mice at Levels Considered Safe for Consumption.* ScienceDaily. https://www.sciencedaily.com/releases/2014/02/140207083619. htm

Bonagura, J. D., & Kirk, R. W. (2000). *Kirk's Current Veterinary Therapy: Small Animal Practice* (13th ed). W. B. Saunders.

Dodds, W. J. (2012). Updated Second Progress Report: Study of Microalbuminuria in Dogs Fed Raw Food Diets. *Dr. Jean Dodds' Pet Health Resource Blog.* https://drjeandoddspethealthresource.tumblr.com/post/35814186 848/raw-diet-affect-on-dog-urine-kidney-renal

Ettinger, S. J., Feldman, E. C., & Côté, E. (Eds.). (2017). *Textbook of Veterinary Internal Medicine: Diseases of the Dog and the Cat* (Eighth edition). Elsevier.

Hand, M. S., Thatcher, C. D., Remillard, R. L., Roudebush, P., Novtony, B. J., & Lewis, L. D. (2010). *Small Animal Clinical Nutrition.* http://www.markmorrisinstitute.org/sacn5_chapters.html

Latimer, K. S., Duncan, J. R., & Prasse, K. W. (2011). *Duncan & Prasse's Veterinary Laboratory Medicine: Clinical Pathology* (5th ed). Wiley-Blackwell.

Lees, G. (2005). Inherited Kidney Diseases in Dogs and Cats. *Tufts' Canine and Feline Breeding and Genetics Conference.* https://www.vin.com/doc/?id=6694800

Osborne, C. A. D., PhD, Davis, L. S., BA, MS, Sanna, J., BS, Unger, L. K., CVT, & O'Brien, T., D. V. M.,. PhD. (1990). *Urine Crystals in Domestic Animals: Laboratory Identification Guide.* Veterinary Medicine Publishing Co.

Willard, M. D., & Tvedten, H. (Eds.). (2012). *Small Animal Clinical Diagnosis by Laboratory Methods* (5th ed). Elsevier.

Picture Credits

Section 1 Photo by charlesdeluvio

Section 2 Photo by Oscar Sutton

Section 3 Photo by Alvan Nee

Section 5 Photo by Timo Volz

Section 6 Photo by Richard Brutyo

Section 7 Photo by Jamie Street

Section 8 Photo by Austin Wilcox

Section 9 Photo by hang niu

Section 10 Photo by Joséphine Menge

Section 11 Photo by charlesdeluvio

Section 12 Photo by Laura Chouette

Section 13 Photo by Max Ducourneau

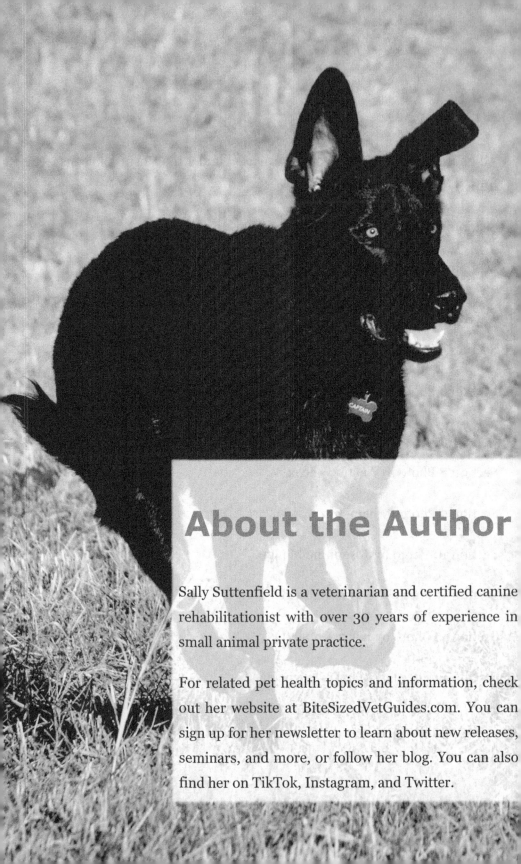

About the Author

Sally Suttenfield is a veterinarian and certified canine rehabilitationist with over 30 years of experience in small animal private practice.

For related pet health topics and information, check out her website at BiteSizedVetGuides.com. You can sign up for her newsletter to learn about new releases, seminars, and more, or follow her blog. You can also find her on TikTok, Instagram, and Twitter.

Made in the USA
Coppell, TX
13 December 2024

42394021R00164